FAMILY DEATH DOULA

SUPPORTING A LOVED ONE THROUGH END OF LIFE

KELLY RUBY HANSON

Published 2025

Cover Design: Marc Gonzales

Editing: Cassandra Van and Ana Abby

Author’s photo courtesy of Cristina Julia

ADVANCE PRAISE

Kelly's wisdom and compassion guide the reader through the challenges of supporting a loved one at the end of life as if she's right there in the room with you.

I really appreciated the consistent theme of self-care and the many effective exercises and practices she offers throughout the book.

Everyone who loves someone should read this book.

— BARBARA B, READER WITH AN ELDERLY MOTHER AND A FRIEND APPROACHING THE END OF LIFE

This book is a beautiful, compassionate, and practical guide for anyone facing the end of a loved one's life. With clarity and warmth, Kelly offers self-care practices that bring comfort and steadiness during times of deep emotional strain.

Her exercises are accessible and grounding—not only for moments of grief, but for any challenging season. This is an essential companion for anyone navigating loss while trying to care for themselves along the way.

— DEBORAH ATELLA, BESTSELLING AUTHOR OF *IS THIS JOB MY JAM? THE GUIDE FOR GROWN-UPS WHO STILL DON'T KNOW WHAT THEY WANT TO BE*

An extraordinary and heartfelt guide, this book is a gift to anyone walking alongside a loved one at the end of life. What stood out most to me was the author's ability to shift gracefully between roles—death doula, daughter, friend—illuminating the many ways we show up for others in their final days. The writing is warm, accessible, and deeply human. The reflective exercises are thoughtfully crafted and sure to be invaluable for caregivers, family members, and patients alike. As a fellow death doula, I especially appreciated the clarity with which the emotional layers of each role were explored. This book is not only a practical resource but a compassionate companion for the journey ahead.

— SITARA TRUMBULL, DEATH DOULA

Brilliant. Clear. Pragmatic. A powerful guide.

Early on Kelly tells us: "What you will learn in this book will build up your internal resources to use in times of need, along with external practices for you to help support your loved one." She fulfills this promise with gentle compassion, a weave of personal stories, and a bevy of pragmatic tools.

Compelling and easy to read, this book will leave you with a richer, deeper understanding of the process of navigating the death journey of a loved one - and your role in it.

A huge contribution to a very complex process.

— ROBIN WINN, MA, LMFT, BESTSELLING AUTHOR, FOUNDER OF AWAKENING THROUGH HUMAN DESIGN

Kelly Ruby Hanson's 'Supporting A Loved One Through End Of Life' offers profound relief by assuring us that there is no perfect way to navigate this sacred journey—only your authentic way. Her gentle wisdom creates space for the full complexity of the human experience while providing comprehensive practical guidance for everything from day-to-day caregiving to navigating difficult conversations and emotional landscapes. The wealth of actionable tools and information serves as a compassionate roadmap during one of life's most challenging passages, offering insights that I found valuable even though I have not yet personally experienced this journey. For anyone supporting a dying loved one, this book is a hand reaching out across the darkness, providing both specific guidance and the comforting assurance that meaningful connection remains possible even in our most vulnerable moments.

— CHARLOTTE FRIBORG, BESTSELLING AUTHOR & COACH FOR WORKING MOMS

For Leland, Lowell, AJ, and Johnathan-
To the ones who made me an aunt…

Thank you for gifting me with new ways to see the world,
for receiving my love, and for encouraging me to make the world a better place.
May the world hold you as softly as I do in my heart.

To Bud and Todd, for showing how even small exchanges can make lasting impacts on others. May your stories continue to be told.

CONTENTS

FOREWORD

I met Kelly through a mutual friend several years ago when I was still actively processing my grief from the loss of my 10-month-old son in 2014. The truth is, our society does a very poor job of talking about death and dying openly, let alone in a healthy, helpful way. Although my exposure to death was generally greater than that of my peers given my status as both a preacher's kid growing up and then as a clergy spouse, each successive personal loss I experienced, taught me how little I knew, let alone understood, about grief and loss. When I suddenly found myself navigating these processes as a 38-year-old post-partum primary caregiver, I felt overwhelmed and unequipped. I struggled to keep my head above water to stay employed as a lawyer and be present as a spouse while caring for my infant son, my 3-year-old, and myself.

During my work with Kelly, I realized that that the work of a death doula is valuable both long before and long after someone's active dying phase.

In these pages, Kelly has distilled her knowledge, experience, and expertise into an accessible guide that creates the necessary space for having more open and helpful conversations around death and dying. Whether discussing issues related to caring for the physical and mental health needs of both the caregiver and the dying loved one, or more practical matters related to paperwork or end-of-life desires and expectations, this book is like having a calm, non-anxious presence with you to help get through a tough moment or ask the right question. I can attest to both the value and the truth of the advice and guidance found within these pages because I learned it the hard way on my own journey.

The utility of this book lies in the coupling of its valuable information and insight with simple practices and exercises. These activities can be done at any point throughout the journey to help reconnect with our loved ones or ourselves and have the potential to make the experience smoother, easier, and more meaningful.

Life and death each unfold in their own way, in their own time. But neither exists without the other. Each leaves its impression on and shapes the other, over and over. This book is a much-needed tool to help us incorporate the difficult conversations around death and dying into our daily living. By doing so, when the time comes for our loved ones to transition from the physical plane, we can be present and offer the gift of ourselves. This is the beautiful gift that Kelly offers us within these pages, and I am so grateful.

— MARY CATHERINE HOBSON, AUTHOR OF
WEATHERED HEARTS

INTRODUCTION: THE SPACE BETWEEN

Sitting at the bedside of a cherished person who is dying brings a kaleidoscope of ever-changing experiences that range from heartbreaking to heart-opening. And the world does not do well in supporting this journey. I remember driving down the street doing something that would have been totally normal in my day when my mom was dying. Stopped at a traffic light, I looked around at the other drivers and thought, "Don't you know my mother is dying?!?!? How can you go about your day when she is leaving me, driving as though nothing has changed?" The light turned green, the thought quieted, and I went on with my errand.

Yet everything had changed. My world was simultaneously standing still and spinning out of control while everyone else's continued at its regular pace. The people who knew about my situation asked about her and how my family was doing, but even those people seemed to want to hurry me through the experience. Their discomfort in talking about death, illness, and maybe their memories of losing someone they loved colored our conversations. And it left me feeling unsupported. It lessened my ability to be present with my mom during her dying time and made my grieving process after her death more complicated.

I assume that since you are reading this book, you are facing a similar situation now—a loved one is dying, and it has set your world spinning in all the wrong directions, leaving you feeling off-balance, out of control, and as though time operates differently. When my mom was diagnosed with lung cancer, the last three months of her life felt like three years. It was hard for me to keep my internal focus on anything but her—was she okay, was she in pain, did she need different care—all while my external focus appeared to operate as normal. Just as you might be doing now with your loved one, I worked, cared for my children, and ran our lives, all while dealing with the logistics and emotions surrounding my mom's end of life.

When a loved one is dying, it may feel as though your world is stopping, but that does not mean the world actually stops. That is one cruelty in this process—you are not given adequate time and space to face what you are experiencing. Even if you were, it probably would not be enough.

WHY I WROTE THIS BOOK

Few people are able to face these types of conversations with a sense of ease and willingness to face the "is" of the moment... This *is* happening, your loved one *is* dying, and surviving this journey feels as though it *is* impossible...

But it is possible. And it is possible to survive your loved one's end-of-life journey without bypassing all the hard parts while offering the best support to them that you can. What that looks like is different for every person. That is what this book is for. It is here for you to read, in the timing that is right for you, to gain strength, support, introspection, some tools, and maybe occasionally a distraction from the hard work of supporting your loved one in their dying journey in a way that reminds you that you can and will survive this.

MY STORY

What is the lesson in this pain? I remember sitting in a Panera, eating my soup and salad, when I read this line in a personal growth book. It was a beautiful May day. Maybe it was April. Time was not moving normally then. My mom was sick. She was more than sick; she was dying. She had been diagnosed with stage IV lung cancer at the end of March. Time moved both fast and slow while we waited for answers, waited to make more decisions, and waited for what we did not want to happen.

The question the book asked made me feel sick. It made me angry. I put down my spoon, picked up my things, and left without cleaning my table. I never did that. The author asked what I could learn from my mother's terminal illness and death at the wrong moment. Finding life lessons in my family's situation was not at the front of my mind. Surviving was. At that time, my main goal was to help my mom get through the end of her life with as little fear and discomfort as possible because what I really wanted- to have my mom not die – I could not have. And I needed to be able to do this while navigating the complications that made up our relationship. So, to ask what lessons I could find in what we were going through enraged me. I wanted to scream, kick over the table, and cry all at the same time. The emotions I felt were not really about the question. They were about how soon I would lose my mom and how little control I had over this. My mom was dying, and since I could not prevent her death, I wanted to help her not be afraid or in pain.

At this point in my life, I had family members who had died- four grandparents, an aunt with leukemia, an uncle from a heart attack, and distant elderly relatives. There were the friends who died young, one in a car crash at 20 and another from a rarc form of cancer in her 30s. Not to mention the many deaths I had experienced at work as a surgical technologist at a level-one trauma hospital. Also, being from a small town, attending funerals was a common activity in my family because if you were not related to the person who died, then you were family friends. My father had the forethought to have my sister, and I help plan our grandmother's funeral to teach us how to do it because we would be doing it for our parents one day. He did not know that day would come much sooner than any of us expected.

Even though I had lost family members who were dear to me and had been on countless surgical teams where the patient did not make it, I had never felt as close to the person who was dying. The relationships I had with my grandparents and aunt were extremely close. We spent a lot of quality time together and shared many wonderful experiences. The closeness I felt with my mom when she was given her diagnosis was maybe that of a protector, an advocate... no, it was that of a companion. Unlike my other family members or my patients, the moment my mom told me she was dying, I decided that I would support her in ways I had not been there for others. Thinking back on it now, maybe my mom's death was the first time I blended the roles I played in caring for my family members in their dying times with the roles I played in the patient deaths at the hospital. With my family, I had a shared history; we spent more time together, and there was story-sharing, laughing, crying, and love. With the patients at the hospital, I had skilled effort, educated responses to problems, professionalism, and compassion. I had never bathed a family member after their death, but I had washed many patients after theirs. I had never been a part of creating values-based care plans with my patients, but I had with my loved ones.

My mom's terminal diagnosis and end-of-life journey would be the first time I would weave together the strengths I relied on at work as a healthcare professional with the ones I held in my family. Without knowing it, this experience would be the first time I would begin using death doula skills. I had no formal training in helping someone at the end of their life. I only had the desire to help my mom, my family, and myself.

At the time of my mom's illness and death, I was working full-time and raising two small kids with my husband. I tried my hardest to not allow any of those things to negatively impact each other, but they did. I accomplished what I had set out to do, support my mom so she would not be afraid or have pain. It was not easy, and my life suffered for it, but I survived, and my family survived. Showing up for my mom in her dying time was worth it. It was healing for our relationship and our extended family. But I remember wishing back then that I had some type of support for me while I sat at the bedside while my mom lay in the bed.

Remember how I said earlier that time moves differently when we experience illnesses and a loved one's dying time? Part of me wants to believe that I can make time operate differently. By writing this book, I would like to think that I can travel back to the time when my mom was dying and give the young woman that I was then the support and guidance in these pages to help her know that there is no perfect way to help someone who is dying. I would tell her that the best thing she could do would be to show up however she could and be present with her mom. I would also like to think that the words on these pages will aid you, the reader, while you sit at your loved one's bedside as they do the hard work of progressing through the end of their life. Ultimately, the words and actions that we offer to our loved ones at the end of life are less important than the presence we provide for them. Let me help you be there for them.

COLLEEN'S STORY: FINDING HER WAY

Reaching my hand across the table, not quite touching her hand, I asked, "Has anybody told you what is happening?" My friend leaned back, scrunching her eyebrows in a sad way that let me know that she wasn't sure what I was asking about and also that she knew exactly what I was saying.

I asked, "Have the doctors said anything?"

Let me pause here and go back a bit to give you some context for this story. My friend Colleen had started posting on social media in the spring about her mom, Renee's breast cancer returning. Her mom's treatments, the tasks involved with taking her to appointments, arranging financial matters, and dealing with her mom's moodiness were topics of her posts mixed in with her usual life adventures. Our friendship was a bigger part of our lives when her mom was first diagnosed with breast cancer years ago. We were neighbors who were included in each other's family gatherings. Our daughters were born a month apart and were each other's first friends. Because of our close friendship and my working in surgery, I was able to support Colleen in a way that no one else could during her mom's first cancer journey by explaining surgical procedures and what questions to ask the doctors. I also knew what food her family liked, so I showered them with love and support by cooking for them. Years had passed since Renee's first diagnosis. Colleen and I both moved to different neighborhoods, and our friendship moved to the periphery. We no longer saw each other regularly, but we never lost the understanding we had of one another. So, when Colleen's posts became more focused on her mom's care and less on her own life, I understood that my friend was struggling. There was an underlying hum to her words that I understood as a death doula. My actions at the time were to offer words of support on her posts and keep watch on how things unfolded. At this point, Colleen and I did not get together anymore. I was no longer working in surgery and was a death doula. I had no plans to step into her family's circumstances, but life has a way of intervening to put us where we need to be. I can't remember exactly what Colleen shared that caused me to reach out to her, but I texted and asked if she would like to meet to talk about her mom. Soon. She gladly agreed to meet me. We quickly set up a time and place.

When I trained as a death doula, I did so intending to work with people who had terminal diagnoses, life-limiting illnesses, those in the late stages of life, and anyone who was interested in planning for a future we will all meet. I did not expect that life would take my work in the direction away from helping the person lying in the bed and focus it instead on the person sitting at the bedside, but here I am.

I looked at Colleen with the softest face I could muster after listening to her share about her mom's last couple of months, along with what options for treatment were available, and said, "Your mother is dying. Has anyone told you that?" I did not say this as a medical professional looking at her mom's medical charts. I am no doctor. In my healthcare career, it was not in my scope of practice to inform people when someone was dying. I was not there to tell my friend when or how her mom would die. I was there to speak the words no one was coming out and saying. I was there as a friend and death doula. Maybe a medical professional did say specifically that her mom was terminal, but that is not what

Colleen was showing that she or her siblings heard. Because of the nature of our friendship and how we had been with each other in years past, I felt comfortable speaking to Colleen this way. I do not go around making a habit of telling people the "truths" I think I see in their situation without their permission. If I did, I would learn that often I was wrong.

I waited, watched, and listened to what my friend was sharing about her mom. I saw Colleen floundering—unsure of what the right thing to do was or how to handle her mom's care, as the only child living in the same area. Colleen felt alone and stressed in trying to help her mom make decisions, decisions that were going to dictate what the end of her mom's life would look like. I could see that Colleen was struggling and was not able to voice that the choices that needed to be made were ones about her mom's dying time. Maybe this was because it was hard for her to accept that her mom was going to die. Maybe it was because she was the only family member present to help. Maybe it was because no one spoke the words so clearly to her.

Either way, I was not telling Colleen something that she did not already know.

I cannot say for sure what my friend got out of the conversation we had that afternoon, but I can say the focus of her mom's care changed. I offered to go and speak with her mom as a death doula to have conversations that Renee may have been unwilling to have with her daughter. Colleen found a way to get her mom into a live-in hospice and helped her stepdad come up with a plan for himself after his wife's death. Her siblings came home and had their last visits with their mom. They had all thought her passing was a long time away. Once everyone - Colleen, her siblings, and her mom- accepted that it was, in fact, happening now, Renee soon took her last breath, surrounded by Colleen, her two granddaughters, and her son-in-law. It was as though once everyone stopped fighting the idea that this time there was no beating cancer, Renee was able to feel her physical pain was controlled enough for her to relax into doing the work of dying. And Colleen was able to do the work of supporting her mom to die.

WHO THIS BOOK IS FOR

This book is for anyone sitting at the bedside of a dying loved one, whether that person is a parent, spouse, sibling, child, friend, or other family member. It's for you if:

- You're feeling overwhelmed by the enormity of supporting someone through their final days.
- You want to be present and supportive but aren't sure how.
- You're trying to balance your own grief with the practical aspects of caregiving.
- You're looking for ways to make this time meaningful despite its difficulty.
- You need support for yourself as you provide support for someone else.

I've written this for you to read in the timing that's right for you—whether that's in small doses between caregiving tasks, during quiet moments at the bedside, or when you need a moment of respite. My hope is that these pages will provide strength, support, introspection, practical tools, and occasionally a compassionate distraction from the hard work of supporting your loved one in their dying journey.

HOW THIS BOOK IS STRUCTURED

Throughout these pages, you will find various tools designed to help you navigate both the emotional and physical landscape of caregiving, particularly during a loved one's end-of-life journey.

Coping Exercises provide comfort, grounding, and emotional regulation, offering support in moments of stress and anxiety. These will help you resource yourself so you're better equipped to face the demands of supporting your loved one.

Pause and Reflect Exercises invite you to slow down and process your feelings, giving you space to acknowledge your emotions and gain insight without rushing.

Writing Reflections encourages exploration through guided prompts, allowing you to express difficult thoughts and create a personal record of your experiences.

Connection Exercises focus on fostering meaningful interactions with your loved one and others, whether through shared moments, meaningful gestures, or creating lasting memories.

The book also includes personal stories from my work, time as a volunteer, and my life. Together, these practices and stories provide various ways to engage with the complexities of supporting your loved one at the end of life, allowing you to reflect, process, and connect in ways that honor both your own needs and your loved one's dying journey.

WHAT YOU WILL TAKE AWAY

I can't promise that this book will make the process of supporting your dying loved one easy—nothing can do that. But I can promise that these pages will help you:

- Find grounding techniques when emotions feel overwhelming.
- Develop a toolkit of responses for difficult moments.
- Discover ways to create meaningful connections during this time.
- Honor both your loved one's journey and your own needs.
- Recognize that imperfection is part of this process.
- Feel less alone in your experience.

You may have heard of the collectivist idea that it takes a village to raise a child. Well, it is my thought that it also takes a village to holistically support someone at the end of their life. Yes, there are many hands-on tasks that are required when caring for a dying person, like changing bedding and managing medications, which rely on physical people. However, there are also other energetic tasks that can be supportive of the dying person and those in their circle. Then, there are the ways in which you can resource yourself so you are better equipped to face the demands of supporting your loved one. This is where the Coping Exercises will help you.

Helping someone through their dying process is not easy. This is where you need to rely on your village – the community of people, whether they are hired professionals, family caregivers, neighbors, or whoever... These are your people's resources. They can be near and far. Their location will influence the help they can provide you. They are able to perform tasks like doing laundry, providing medical care, reading to your loved one… the list goes on and on. The other parts of the village include things like prayer groups, online forums where you can find people in similar situations as you to share with and ask questions, websites like CaringBridge where you can share information one time instead of speaking your loved one's story an exhausting number of times, and resources like this book. These first two groups of resources are your external resources.

In this book, we will also cover the internal resources that will help you navigate your loved one's dying journey. These will allow you to find anchors to hold onto when you need something to help you hold your head above water. Some days, supporting someone at the end of life is like swimming in quiet, calm waters, and other days, you will find yourself in rough seas. Everyone's dying process is unique. I wish I could map out for you how your loved one's dying time will go, but I cannot. I can guide and teach you about what you might see and experience, but I cannot give you the certainty of knowing exactly how it will go. What I can do and will hopefully do in this book is to provide you with a life raft when you need it. Think of the words in this book as a stand-in for my physical presence sitting beside you as you do the difficult work of helping your loved one live out the remainder of their life.

You are there for them. I am here for you.

The journey ahead won't be easy, but with support, it can be meaningful, authentic, and even healing. As we move forward through these pages together, remember that there is no perfect way to help someone who is dying. The best thing you can do is show up however you can and be present with your loved one. Ultimately, the words and actions we offer to our loved ones at the end of life are less important than the presence we provide. Let me help you be there for them.

PART I

BEGINNING THE JOURNEY

1

UNDERSTANDING YOUR ROLE

Robert, or Rob as I came to call him, and I first met when I walked through his hospital room door. Our introduction was quiet and quick as the volunteer I was relieving updated me on Robert's status. She, like me, had come to sit at Rob's bedside because he was dying, and no one from his family was able to attend what were thought to be his last hours of life.

A friend of his had stopped in a couple of times after Rob was admitted to the hospital, but the friend never stayed long. The times I saw the friend, he seemed sad and uncomfortable, unsure of what he could do to support someone dying in the hospital. I made up a little story in my mind that the friend brought in the book of fiction I saw sitting on the shelf in the room and the pillows that were not standard-issue hospital pillows for Robert.

As I looked around the room, I noticed that Robert had a tele-sitter, also known as a virtual sitter. This remote patient monitoring device is used when patients in hospitals are at risk of getting out of bed and falling or when the patient's care requires a constant watchful eye that our current medical staffing models do not allow for. There is nothing inherently wrong with using this device; it is yet another tool in the medical team's arsenal of monitoring systems used to improve patient care and ease the workload of overburdened staff. As a former hospital employee, I understand the need for technology such as this, but that night, seeing the machine in Robert's room made me feel sad because it felt like a confirmation that he had no one sitting at his bedside to support him.

This man had received a cancer diagnosis a while back before coming to the hospital. It was not shared with me whether he had received treatment for it or not. The role that I was playing in Robert's end-of-life journey did not warrant my knowing the specifics of his medical history. I was not there as a healthcare provider. I was there as a volunteer sitting vigil with him, attending to his dry mouth, alerting the nurse when his pain became too much, and shifting pillows to help ease his discomfort. In the many hours that I sat with Robert, I sometimes read quietly to myself. Other times, I held his hand, I moistened his mouth, and when he spoke, I tried to make sense of his words.

As I watched over Robert, there were countless times when his breathing changed or stopped altogether, and I would think, "Is this it?" When the CNA came in to take Robert's vitals, I told her that they were probably going to be bad. She looked confused and concerned by my words. I told her about Rob's breathing patterns as she pushed the button to record his blood pressure and oxygen levels. Seeing the results, she looked at me and quickly called his nurse, who I can only assume informed the young professional that the patient was at the end of his life, would not have good vital signs, and that they were not giving any interventions to improve them. They were only providing comfort care as he transitioned from life to death.

Eventually, because Robert's dying process was taking longer than anticipated, he was able to be moved into a hospice facility. This is when my time with him ended. I will never know the end of his story or if anyone was at his bedside with him when he died, but I can say that everyone involved in his care was part of a village of caregivers. Some of us were healthcare providers, some were nonmedical chaplain volunteers, and others were friends. No matter how much time we as individuals spent with Robert, we all permeated his dying time with compassionate care and energy.

Even the people in his life who were not present at his bedside could energetically help Rob during his dying process. That thought may be a stretch for you, but I was taught, and I believe, that we are all connected in ways beyond our understanding. You may think of it as offering thoughts and prayer or sending energy, or maybe that we are all symbiotically connected to each other in unseen ways, like the mycorrhizal networks that connect mushrooms to each other and the plants around them. Whatever your belief, it is not the purpose of this book to get into a discussion on naming what the connections between us are. The purpose is to offer ways to utilize the connections to help you survive the time you spend supporting your loved one's dying time.

WHAT IS A DEATH DOULA?

As you move forward with the awareness that you have decided to play an active role in supporting your loved one as they live out the remainder of their life, you can begin to select aspects of a death doula you would like to take on. To begin, let me clarify how the work a death doula performs is defined so you can decide what death doula skills you would like to practice during your loved one's dying time.

> *A death doula is a practitioner who provides nonmedical care for individuals transitioning to death and their families. This care encompasses the emotional, mental, physical, spiritual, and practical needs of their clients.*

The time frame in which a doula may work with someone can range from end-of-life pre-planning during times of health, to support after a terminal diagnosis, through the active dying process, and into the bereavement period. The profession of death doula is not regulated. The scope of practice for a death doula can be wide.

CORE PRINCIPLES OF DEATH DOULA PRACTICE

Compassionate Presence

First and foremost, as a death doula, I enter the dying space, holding kindness and compassion in my heart. Being a death doula is open practice—open hands and open heart, willing to receive and give what is needed. It is not an unkind practice, so don't be unkind to yourself.

When I trained as a death doula, I noticed immediately how altruistic my teachers were. This in no way is meant to say that people who are death doulas put others' needs before their own. Instead, they are trained in the ability to be well-informed about their own internal experience while having an understanding and curiosity for the other person's experience.

I call this balance the fifty-fifty: half of the doula's attention goes to self-awareness—monitoring their own internal and external state—and the other half to being present with the client.

A personal example of this is the story of Robert. He

happened to have the same cancer diagnosis as my Aunt Rita. When I learned of their shared diagnosis and saw how Robert's time at the hospital was full of pain, I had to take a moment to center myself. I had to take a deep breath, feel my back touching up against my chair, acknowledge my fears that my aunt's experience could potentially be like Robert's, and then let it all exist. I did not try to change my feelings and worries as I came back to see the person before me. Life is full of complexities. You can be present for someone and still have thoughts about yourself.

Building a Circle of Support

Second, as a death doula, I work with the people who surround the dying person to create their circle. This circle or community becomes a family that helps to sustain the dying person. This family or circle can be made up of people who are united by biology, by spoken commitments, by shared community, and by volunteer or hired professionals. It is made up of all individuals drawn into the experience of the dying person. They need not be physically present to have an impact in the dying space. Support comes in many forms, especially for a person at the end of their life and those who are physically supporting them.

Creating a Healing Space

Other aspects of the work a death doula performs are to promote and accept positive and negative feelings as they authentically listen to and witness others' stories. They allow space for emotions that come up instead of rushing through them. Doulas foster sensitive awareness by nurturing other's beliefs and practices. Through their work, they create a healing environment for the physical and spiritual parts of a person that respects individual dignity. This environment is what I professionally call the deathbed ecosystem.

The dying space or deathbed ecosystem should be co-created with the doula, the dying person, and those in their circle. It should set the dying person at ease. The work that a doula performs brings the essence of hope into a time that may be full of undesired outcomes while facing the truth of the situation. This is not hope for a cure but instead hope of comfort, courage, love, personal growth, happiness for one's family, or possibly a better understanding of the mysteries at the end of life.

Serving someone in their dying time is based on developing healing, helping, and trusting relationships. This is done by accepting what happens every day for the dying person. It is not the job of the doula to heal all past experiences or to explicitly prevent future hurts. Their work often has this impact, but they are not therapists trained to focus exclusively on this type of work. They do, however, operate with an understanding of the complex nature of relationships and how they can impact the dying space.

Death doulas can also assist with the practical physical and planning needs of the dying person. They use creative, scientific problem-solving skills to address individual needs. One of the biggest talents of doulas is the practice of remaining open to the mysteries that show up in the dying space.

Adapting Death Doula Skills for Your Role

A good portion of the work a death doula does starts with their relationship with themselves. Saying you have to do self-development work while supporting your loved one at the end of life is a big ask. Supporting your loved one does not have to feel like a therapy session, but learning a few simple therapeutic tools can help you feel more grounded and better prepared for the journey.

I want to equip you with tools and knowledge so you survive the experience of assisting your loved ones during their dying time, not make this a graded homework assignment for you. If you can learn how to mobilize the available resources needed to manage aspects of the dying process, then maybe your loved one and you will not suffer too many decreases in the quality of your lives.

What I want you to learn is how to cope with the demands of caregiving for someone at the end of life and to know when those demands have exceeded your perceived resources so you can adjust to get more help or change how care is provided. I also want you to understand that every death is different. There are parts to the dying process that do not deviate from one death to another. Only the timeline of events does.

Dying is hard work. It requires effort from the individual. Some deaths appear easier than others. Different disease processes, chronic illnesses, and living conditions can impact how a person moves through their dying time.

Your Unique Position in the Dying Circle

While you will be learning the skills of a death doula to bolster the ways you show up for your loved one, you will still be who you were in your relationship with them. Your role or title will not change. You will not have solely a professional connection with them that a working death doula has with their clients. You have a history with the dying person that extends beyond this phase of their life, and so do many of the other people in the dying circle.

In this book, you will learn ways to compassionately hold the complicated relational interactions that can show up in the dying space. I can speak from experience and say that it is different to companion another at the end of life when they are tied to you through years of shared experiences than it is with someone that you are professionally supporting.

An example of this is The way I interact with my aunt Rita around the topic of her diagnosis and end of life compared to the way I interacted with Robert. My aunt does not see me as a professional coming to guide her. I am her niece, who happens to work with dying and grieving people. With Robert, I was a professional who spent a limited time at his bedside, providing comfort and support. Why is it important to understand the differences between those roles? Because no matter how many skills you learn, your loved one may not want you to step out of the existing relational roles you have had.

The Inner Journey of Caregiving

As you navigate this dual role—being both a loved one and a caregiver—your internal landscape will inevitably shift and change. While you sit at the bedside of your loved one, there is a deeply personal journey that unfolds within you during this time. This is another area where death doulas receive specific preparation, and understanding it can help you maintain your balance during challenging moments.

The responsibility of caring for a loved one during their dying time takes place as you witness changes to their body, abilities, and mind. The realization that there will be a future where your loved one is absent may also come to mind. When this does happen and your mind or emotions stray, be kind to yourself. Another contemplation that can come up when supporting someone at the end of their life is the thought of your own mortality. Death doula education includes deep considerations about a student's own mortality.

It is a part of the work. You do not have to use your loved one's dying time as an exercise to consider your own mortality, though. Doing so may add too much to your already heavy burden. You certainly can, but it is not a requirement. Just know that the feelings and behaviors that come up in the dying space may be others' or your own reactions to the apprehension concerning one's own impermanence.

This awareness—that your thoughts about mortality are natural but not mandatory to explore deeply right now—is another tool you can carry forward from death doula practice. Your primary role is to be present for your loved one in whatever way feels authentic to your relationship while also maintaining enough self-care to sustain you through this journey.

The Purpose of This Book

It is my goal in the following chapters to provide you with an understanding of the dimensions involved in the dying process, foster your feeling of empowerment by teaching you tools and techniques for being with your loved one, and guide you in ways that increase your comfort level with participating in your loved one's end of life.

Use the information in this book in ways that best serve you. Some concepts and practices will appeal to you, but others may not. Take what works and discard what does not. Think of all the information in this book as an invitation to show up and be with another human being as they live out the remainder of their life. There is no right or wrong way to progress through this challenging process.

What you will learn in this book will build up your internal resources to use in times of need, along with external practices for you to help support your loved one. Our mind likes it when it has something to work on. I am going to provide you with ideas about being in relationship and death doula skills to occupy your mind, which will give your heart time to catch up to what is happening in your loved one's life. There will be tools you learn that you can apply in the immediate time, and there will be layers of concepts to hold onto to help you process this journey later.

Lastly, I hope that this book serves as a good stand-in for me and that its words leave you feeling supported and capable—because you are.

As we continue through this book, we'll explore specific skills and approaches you can adapt from death doula practice to support your loved one. Remember that your presence—your willingness to simply be there—is perhaps the most powerful gift you can offer during this time. Everything else builds upon that foundation.

COPING EXERCISE: The Fifty-fifty Awareness Practice

Develop the skill of balanced attention between yourself and your loved one.

Purpose: To maintain awareness of your own internal experience while remaining present and attentive to your loved one, preventing emotional overwhelm while ensuring quality care.

Time needed: 2-3 minutes initially; practice regularly to develop this skill

Instructions:

1. Begin by taking a deep breath and noticing where your body makes contact with its support (chair, floor, etc.).
2. Gently scan your internal landscape, acknowledging any emotions, physical sensations, or thoughts arising within you. Don't try to change them—simply notice.
3. Name these experiences to yourself: "I'm feeling anxious," "My shoulders are tense," "I'm worried about what comes next."
4. Now, with this self-awareness as your foundation, turn your attention to your loved one.
5. Observe them with curiosity and care, noticing their expressions, breathing, positioning, and any cues they may be giving.
6. Continue to maintain this dual awareness—50% attuned to your own experience, 50% attuned to theirs.
7. If you notice yourself becoming overwhelmed by either your emotions or theirs, gently return to your breath and physical sensations as an anchor.
8. Remember: You can be present for someone while still having thoughts and feelings about yourself.

Reflection: How does maintaining awareness of your own experience change how you interact with your loved one? What do you notice about your capacity to be present when you're not trying to suppress your own feelings?

2

THE RELATIONAL TAPESTRY

One day, when I was 8, I was sitting in my room with its soft yellow walls in front of a loom that stood upright, pulling yarn over and under the strings. One after another, I wove the yarn, occasionally stopping to push the string down with my weaving comb or to tie a knot and start a new color.

As I have struggled to explain the importance of personal relationships and their histories in the dying space, this memory came back to me. It was comforting, and it calmed my mind, helping me come into the presence of my thoughts. That was when I realized that my childhood hobby of weaving was similar to how relationships interact.

In both cases, you start with a structure. For relationships, let's start with a family and ancestors. The ancestors are like the loom itself, providing the foundation that holds everything together - unseen but essential. The loom stands steady, its frame woven with the threads of the past, offering support on which everything else is built.

The warp strings—those long, steady threads that run through the loom—represent the qualities and connections that make up a person. These threads form the backbone of who someone is, and as they are woven around, they build the fabric of the individual's identity. The loom holds these warp strings in place, much like how our relationships with family and ancestors hold us steady in the world.

It is in this sacred space where the foundation of relationships is built and hearts begin to intertwine. When you look at a completed piece of woven tapestry, you do not see the structure that supported it when it was being created, just as you don't see the structure that created an individual. You don't see the ancestors and experiences that shaped a person, just as you don't see the loom and warp strings holding together the fibers.

Energetic connections in relationships, like connections in the weaving process, are often hidden—only their visible patterns remain.

The relational tapestry is an intricate weave of the connections and relationships that join the fabric of your life. In it are threads that represent different people, your identity to those people, feelings you have about them, and experiences you share with them. Each thread is a different color, maybe even a different texture. This weave is made up of physical and energetic ties that bind you to your loved one with different colored threads. Not only that, but your loved one has their own unique tapestry, too.

As a weaver uses the shuttle to pass between the warp strings, relationships work in much the same way. The shuttle moves between the threads, carrying the weft—the interactions, the connections—that fill the space. Every encounter is like the passage of the shuttle, weaving together the fabric of a person's life and relationships.

The give and take in relationships— the kindnesses, the challenges, the growth— creates tension in the threads. This tension is not an obstacle but a force that creates depth and resilience. Tension is what makes the tapestry rich with complexity, where colors and textures blend and new patterns emerge. As the threads are woven, the tension between them strengthens the piece, shaping it into something beautiful and enduring. Similarly, the tensions we encounter in relationships help shape and define the tapestry of our connections.

Over time, the pattern emerges. Every exchange, every experience, leaves its mark, like a distinct thread forming a unique pattern. No two relationships are the same; the design is as individual as the people involved. The pattern, visible only as it unfolds, tells the story of who we are, how we've grown, and how we've intertwined with others. And when the tapestry is finished—when a person is fully formed—you see the richness of the design. The final piece reveals not only the individual but all the relationships that have shaped them along the way. The person you know and love is not just who they are in relation to you, but a reflection of countless moments, connections, and experiences. Like a completed tapestry, there are many parts to people, and each thread contributes to the whole.

THE TAPESTRY IN THE DYING SPACE

When you enter your loved one's dying space, you do so as a whole person present with another whole person. Both of you bring your being, your thoughts, feelings, experiences, and relationships to form a tapestry that moves forward and backward in time and experience to include all that you have touched and will ever touch. Life is not static, as people and situations are always changing, which means people are continually weaving their tapestries.

Supporting a loved one during their dying time is stressful. It might help you to have a framework to understand how your relationship with your loved one, both of your life experiences, and your other connections, may influence the time you have left together.

The relational tapestry is an intricate weave of the connections that join the fabric of your life. In it are threads that represent different people, your identity to those people, feelings you have about them, and experiences you share with them. Each thread is a different color, maybe even a different texture. Not only that, but your loved one has their own unique tapestry, too.

It is as though when sitting in a room full of people, there exists an invisible connection between every person's individual tapestries. Some are joined tightly together and solid —similar to how you may have a closer relationship with one sibling over another. Regardless of the quality and strength of the strings, a connection exists. Even when the physical strings are cut in relationships, energetic connections remain.

WHY THE TAPESTRY MATTERS

So what does all this have to do with supporting your loved one in their dying time? And why is it relevant to surviving the experience? It is because every time you interact with someone, you unknowingly interact with their history and life stories. No time demonstrates that more than during the end of someone's life.

How many movies have you seen where family members reveal truths or have healing moments over a parent's deathbed? There are so many because it is *partially* true. There is a raw energy in the space and time when a loved one is dying. It cracks you open and can lead to reconciliation and growth, but that does not mean that every person's death is full of relational healing and connection. Life just does not happen that way.

It is helpful to remember in the dying space that your life experience, values, thoughts, and feelings—your tapestry—bumps up against others' tapestries. Sometimes that can be abrasive.

WHEN TAPESTRIES COLLIDE

An example of this is the unit secretary on the hospital floor where a man I was visiting as a death doula had a change in medical status. The man's family was not ready to embrace the news that he was dying. As I passed the desk, I heard the secretary comment to the man's nurse that the family needed to accept the situation and act swiftly to get care.

My first reaction was to tell her she should be more sensitive. Obviously, the family wasn't ready to face their loved one's end of life. But I understood that the secretary carried her own complicated history that was coloring how she reacted. Her relational tapestry influenced her thoughts and feelings, which affected her behavior. Who knows how many sad stories she had witnessed and what effect they had on her.

Instead, I integrated her and what happened into my own tapestry in order to remind myself that in the dying space, I need to rely on my patience when interacting with the other people present— even with the professionals taking part in the care of the dying person.

Now imagine the tension that might surface when the relational tapestries bumping into one another belong to relatives of the dying person. Consider how those unique stories impact the ways family members interact with each other and the dying loved one. I have seen this tension enough times to know that with some people, anything concerning dying brings out the worst in them. I see this less and less these days, but this theme still crops up every now and again.

Usually, when I do see it now, it is a fleeting exchange that can be mediated by giving the people experiencing the tension space and a place to share their thoughts or questions. What I have learned is that each person in the dying space has a history with the dying person- even the professionals providing care. The histories may be full of beautiful connections that have been easy to integrate or miniature traumas that have been painful to weave together. Either way, all anyone is doing in the dying space is the best they can to cope.

THE COMFORT OF OVERLAPPING TAPESTRIES

Sometimes, relational tapestries layer upon each other and provide comfort like a weighted blanket. Decades ago, long before I entered healthcare or deathcare work, my dad called me to tell me that my grandfather had chosen to not take treatment for his prostate cancer. He also said that my grandpa would die from cancer, and that would be happening sooner than later. I was heartbroken. My aunt Micki, my dad's oldest sister, had just died from a lengthy battle with leukemia, and we had not had time to recover from her death.

I was originally told my grandpa would survive his cancer. That it was very treatable. What I did not know was that because of my aunt's experience, my grandpa chose to not undergo any more treatment. I was devastated. I took to my bed to cry, as that was the only thing I could think of doing.

In the background of the exchange with my dad, my emotions and my reaction was my boyfriend, watching it all play out. You see, he had lost his mother to a terrible accident when he was in sixth grade. The building her bridal shop was in collapsed and killed her. This loss was a huge part of his relational tapestry. He knew grief. He took that understanding and did not speak. All he did was lie behind me, holding me as I sobbed. It was as though he understood that he could not fix my grandfather's cancer. He could not prevent my grandpa's death, but in my moments of sadness, he could be present with me and let me have my emotions fully.

His relational tapestry rested upon mine like a weighted blanket, calming my thoughts so I could survive the heartbreak of the moment.

BEYOND PHYSICAL COMMUNICATION

Another way to view the relational tapestry is to see that even when your loved one is no longer able to communicate in their dying time, the connection still exists. There is an unseen thread that joins the two of you that does not need to be validated by speaking the connection out loud.

Starting to see your relationship with your dying loved one this way may help stretch the limitations of your relationship. It offers you the potential to continue your relationship after your loved one reaches the end of their life by transforming some of your grief and loss into connection. There is no way that the idea of a relational tapestry will take away all of your sadness, but it may add a little weight like a blanket, providing a small measure of comfort to you.

The tapestry of relationships is sacred. It does not exist within the limits of time or space. It is not a physical object. Rather, it can be an embodied metaphor that acts as an extension of who you are and those who have touched your life.

Unlike mixing ingredients in baking or paints in art, the metaphorical threads of those who have touched your life don't lose their properties by combining. The colors and flavors of your life and your loved one's life are both separate and intertwined.

Your loved one will always be a part of your tapestry, and you will always be a part of theirs, regardless of whether blood pumps through either of your bodies and oxygen fills your lungs.

JEN'S STORY: TAPESTRIES UNRAVELING AND CONNECTING

It was an unremarkable day. Absolutely normal until the phone call. Jen's brother started the call with his usual "Hey, Sis" opener, to which she casually responded- "what's up?" The words that came next made her feel like she had been punched in the stomach. He simply said, "Sis, I'm dying. I have maybe a year to live if I get treatment. Maybe a few months more..." With that, Jen began walking in two worlds at one time- one where she had to function as though everything and everyone was fine. The other was where her brother was dying.

What made it worse was that her father had died not even a year, maybe two years ago. At that moment, time got funny, and she could not remember clearly the timeline of her loss. All she knew was that she was not over her father's death. She did not think she ever would be, and now, here she was, faced with another potential loss.

When her father was diagnosed with cancer, everyone was so kind. They asked how he was doing and how she was doing. They were generous in their offers of assistance, though at the time, she needed little help. Her father was an effortlessly social man who was prepared for everything without preparing for anything. He was surrounded by friends and family during his illness and his dying time, just like he had been in life.

His presence was a testament to how a person could connect with others, even strangers, in lasting ways. Through these connections, not only was he able to build his network of friends, he was also able to show his children how to do the same – to connect with others in a way that builds a community of support and companionship. His life and death taught Jen how to be self-sufficient while also showing her she could rely on others.

In terms of our relational tapestry concept, Jen's father was a master weaver. The threads he connected throughout his life created a support network that held him during his final days. His tapestry was richly colored with friendships and family bonds, each thread intertwining with countless others. He showed Jen how to weave her own connections, a skill she would need even more as she faced her brother's illness.

Jen's dad's death left a big hole in her heart that had not yet begun to close up, and now, with her brother's impending death, it felt as if that hole would consume her. This is where we see how tapestries can be damaged - threads torn, patterns disrupted. Yet, even in their damaged state, they continue to influence how we engage with the world.

As the days after her brother's diagnosis passed, Jen told more people that he was sick. Her brother was much younger than her dad was when he received his diagnosis. Jen was not sure if that was the reason or if it was that she still felt raw from her father's death, but the way people responded to her was different. It was as though people had finite amounts of patience for her grief, especially in addition to her feelings about her brother's situation.

Here, we see how tapestries collide and sometimes fail to connect. The threads from others' tapestries - their discomfort with death, their limited capacity for supporting ongoing grief - created tension against Jen's tapestry of fresh pain and uncertainty. Where her father's connections had created comfort, these interactions created isolation.

Maybe she had not noticed it when her father was sick, but she saw it now. Pity. When Jen spoke to people about her brother, their expressions changed from shock at the news to pity, then to a small glimmer of thankfulness that it was not them going through this. As her brother progressed, Jen began to recognize another expression on people's faces-avoidance. She learned that people would ask how he was doing, but they did not really want to know. They did not know how to respond to her. They fumbled their words of support. Her family's situation made them uncomfortable.

Jen quickly learned to cut conversations short and save the details of what was happening for a small group of people, but it was hard because the one person she would have normally shared her thoughts with was the person who was sick- her brother.

So there Jen was, left feeling fuzzy, gutted, and alone all at the same time. Trying to live life as normal when it felt anything but. How could she carry on as normal when her head was full of worries about her brother and his children, worries about what he was really thinking… Was he scared? Was he in pain?

Jen was worried about what his illness and death meant for her. Was she going to get sick and die, too? What would happen to their family? Why him? Why now? It was easier for her to stay with the chaos of her thoughts rather than to allow the grief in her heart to open up. Once it opened up, she did not know if it would ever close again and it had to. Jen had to learn to live through feeling gutted inside while still functioning on the outside, and she had to do this all while supporting her brother through the end of his life.

That's where our time together began because in order for Jen to keep one foot in both worlds, she needed at least one person for whom she did not have to edit her experience. She needed one face that would not say, "Please make your answer to my question about your brother quick. Don't tell me anything too uncomfortable."

In the relational tapestry framework, what Jen needed was someone whose threads could intertwine with her damaged tapestry without pulling away. She needed a steady presence who could hold the tension of her grief without breaking. She needed someone who could see the complex pattern of her relationships and honor them all - her relationship with her brother, her father, herself, and her grief.

Jen's brother did not ask for a death doula to work with him; Jen specifically did not ask for a death doula to work with her either. What Jen did ask for was someone who could support her as her brother progressed through his illness, help her to function in her life away from his bedside, and maybe teach her a few things that she could use to help him as he began the process of leaving his physical world behind. Jen needed someone whose face would respond with an unafraid expression, knowing that although the outcome would be difficult, she would make it through this.

CONNECTION PRACTICE: A Loving Touchstone

Create a physical object that carries your love and connection.

Purpose: To establish a tangible symbol of your love that can provide comfort and connection for both you and your loved one.

The time needed: 15-20 minutes for initial preparation; ongoing moments of connection

Instructions:

1. Find a smooth, beautiful stone that feels comforting in your hands.
2. Hold it close to your heart, allowing it to absorb your love and energy.
3. As you hold the stone, silently offer all the loving thoughts and feelings you wish to share with your loved one—those tender expressions of care, even the ones that go unspoken.
4. When the time feels right, bring the stone to your loved one's space. If they are able, encourage them to hold it gently in their hands. If not, place the stone on their bedside table.
5. Allow your loved one to hold the stone as often as they desire, feeling the quiet connection it fosters between you.
6. After your loved one has passed, keep the stone close, a tangible reminder of the love you shared.

Reflection: How does this physical object create a connection between you? What emotions arise when you touch the stone? How might this simple object serve as a bridge between you even when words are difficult to find?

~

COPING EXERCISE: Soothing and Supportive Touch Practice

Use gentle self-touch to calm your nervous system and provide comfort.

Purpose: To ground yourself in moments of stress or overwhelm through intentional, nurturing touch.

Time needed: 5-15 minutes

Instructions:

1. Bring your palms together, noticing the warmth and connection between your hands.
2. Cup your hands in your lap, palms facing up, allowing your body to settle.
3. Move your hands to hover near your heart, feeling the warmth.
4. Gently place one hand on your clavicle (collarbone) area, rubbing or circling with light pressure.
5. Place one hand over the other on your chest, feeling your heartbeat.
6. Use one hand to stroke or make circles on your chest while the other rests.
7. Place one hand on your heart and one on your belly with light pressure.

8. Rest both hands on your belly, feeling the rise and fall of your breath.
9. Place one hand softly on your cheek.
10. Place both hands on each cheek, feeling the warmth.
11. Position one hand on your cheek and one on your forehead.
12. Cross your arms and hug yourself across your chest.
13. Cross your arms and hug around your shoulders.
14. Cross your arms and hug around your belly.
15. Gently stroke your forearms.
16. Return to cupping your hands in your lap.
17. Explore any other gentle touches that feel soothing to you.

Reflection: Which touchpoints felt most calming? How did your body respond to different forms of touch? What changes did you notice in your breathing or tension levels?

PART II

CREATING THE DEATHBED ECOSYSTEM

3

THE DOMAINS OF DYING

When supporting a loved one through the end of life, you enter what might feel like uncharted territory. Yet this space—this final chapter of life—has dimensions and contours that can be understood, navigated, and even transformed into a place of meaning and connection.

THE DEATHBED ECOSYSTEM: A FRAMEWORK FOR UNDERSTANDING

As a death doula, I have found that thinking of the dying process as an "ecosystem" helps both the dying person and their loved ones make sense of what's happening and what's needed. This deathbed ecosystem comprises three essential elements that work together:

> *The Domains of Dying - The different aspects of human experience that need attention during the dying process*

> *End-of-Life Planning - The conversations and decisions that clarify wishes and values*

Creating Sacred Space - The intentional environment that honors the transition

In this chapter, I will cover the domains of dying. Information on end-of-life planning and creating a sacred space will be covered in the next two chapters.

THE DOMAINS OF DYING

Death asks for no specific room requirements or creature comforts. It does not care whether a person is at home or in a facility, but we as people, do. The environment we create around the dying process matters deeply—not just for the comfort of the dying person, but for everyone involved in this profound transition.

Other aspects of the work a death doula performs are to promote and accept positive and negative feelings as they authentically listen to and witness others' stories. They allow space for emotions that come up instead of rushing through them. Doulas foster sensitive awareness by nurturing others' beliefs and practices. Through their work, they create a healing environment for the physical and spiritual parts of a person that respects individual dignity. This environment is what I professionally call the deathbed ecosystem.

As a death doula, setting up a deathbed ecosystem often takes place before a person enters their active dying time with conversations about what the individual's wishes are for the end of life. The conversations are meant to highlight the person's values, how they define the quality of life, what types of care they would like to receive, where they would like to live out the remainder of their life, and whether it is all logistically possible. This work is the heart of creating what I call a values-based care plan for the end of life. This plan sets a clear vision of a person's end-of-life plans and desires. It touches all domains of the dying process by establishing baselines for meeting the individual's physical, emotional, mental, spiritual, and practical needs.

I am going to start off by defining the different domains of needs that present themselves in the deathbed ecosystem, and then we will touch on how to co-create a plan based on meeting those needs with your loved one.

THE PHYSICAL DOMAIN: CREATING COMFORT AND SAFETY

Physical needs are based on human physiology and the physical environment. These needs include the basics when it comes to human survival- food, water, adequate shelter, and clean air to breathe. Physical care of the dying is made up of specific tasks that include but are not limited to attending to your loved one's hygiene, nutrition, skin care, comfort, and the prevention and treatment of symptoms. These needs can be met by formal, professional caregivers such as hospice workers, nurses, or staff at living facilities and by informal, family caregivers.

Also included in this dimension are topics like what type of care a person wants to receive, what physically makes them comfortable, how they want to cope with physical pain or discomfort, and what type of environment they want to be in during the end of their life. This domain is important because it is the area where physical safety is created. Your loved one may be experiencing a loss of bodily control and ability. It can hurt a person's feelings when their body seems to be working against them instead of with them.

The sense of safety created through the physical environment and the awareness that their bodily needs will be attended to by other people and are not a burden will ease the tension that comes up in their dying process. It also helps your loved one to know that any pain or discomfort they experience will be managed. People can be more afraid of pain than they can be of death. We cannot change the fact that, as humans, one day, we will all die, but we can change the fear of abandonment and pain that could happen during a person's dying time.

CONNECTION PRACTICE: A Blanket of Love and Connection

Create a physical token of connection that provides both comfort and meaning.

Purpose: To create a tangible symbol of love and support that can provide physical comfort and emotional reassurance.

Time needed: Initial setup: 1-2 hours; Ongoing additions: 5-10 minutes per person

Instructions:

1. Find a light-colored blanket or sheet, one that can hold the words of care and connection. You may choose to repurpose one from your loved one's home or your own, allowing it to carry the essence of shared memories.
2. Using fabric markers, invite those who have been a part of your loved one's life to write messages of love, support, and well-wishes on the blanket.
3. As you cover your beloved with this blanket, wrap them in the warmth of the heartfelt words and the kindness of those who have touched their life.

4. As visitors come, encourage them to add their own messages to the blanket, continuing to weave a fabric of compassion and connection.

Reflection: How does this physical object create both comfort and connection? What messages seem to bring your loved one the most peace?

THE EMOTIONAL DOMAIN: HONORING FEELINGS AND RELATIONSHIPS

The emotional domain is where feelings reside. It is created through relationships that the dying person has with others and with themselves. There may be events that occurred in your loved one's life prior to their dying time that influence how they cope with their end of life. The same could be said for those who are supporting the dying person. Openness and sensitivity to the feelings and emotions that arise in the dying space are paramount for both your loved one and all that surrounds them.

Now, that does not mean it is your job to become your loved one's therapist. It can mean that you enter into the space and the relationship with your loved one with a heightened awareness that behaviors are often the result of individual strategies for handling daily life. How a person acts is a result of the cumulative lived experiences and the coping mechanisms they learned to deal with those experiences.

Topics included in the emotional dimension include expressed feelings, challenges with feelings, relationship issues, and fears about feeling out of control. The tasks involved in attending to the emotional dimension involve communicating and patience. If your loved one expresses a desire to speak to someone or your intuition tells you it would be beneficial, further assistance in this area can come from therapists, social workers, counselors, spiritual advisors, or confidantes. Even dying people can use mental health tools such as therapy and medications if they are needed. Remember, though, that your loved one may not be open to talking about their internal experience or their life experiences, so do not force the issue. It may be you who needs someone to talk to about the emotional dimension. Do not be afraid to seek help.

WRITING REFLECTION: Grief Journal: A Space for Your Heart's Words

Create a private space to process your emotions throughout this journey.

Purpose: To provide an outlet for exploring feelings that may be difficult to express aloud and to document your experience for later reflection.

Time needed: 5-20 minutes, as often as needed

Instructions:

1. Create a grief journal as a safe, open space where your thoughts, feelings, and experiences can flow without judgment.
2. Begin by writing freely, allowing whatever comes to mind to fill the pages. There's no right or wrong here—whether it's a simple observation or deep, complex emotions.

3. If words feel difficult to find, give yourself permission to scribble or doodle on the page.
4. If free writing doesn't resonate, consider using these prompts:
    - My happiest memory of you is...
    - Something I appreciate about you is...
    - What I miss most about how you were before now is...
    - I am handling your dying time by...
    - What I appreciate about your current care is...
    - What I wish I could change about your current care is...
    - What feelings do I have about my loved one's dying time?
    - What are my biggest concerns about their dying?
    - What are the most important things I would like my loved ones to know about our relationship before they pass away?
    - What can I learn from this experience?
    - What does this experience make me want to prioritize in my life?
    - In what ways can I support my loved one?

Reflection: How does writing change your relationship with difficult emotions? Are there patterns in what brings you comfort or distress?

THE MENTAL DOMAIN: PRESERVING LEGACY AND MEANING

The mental domain of the dying process is where a dying person's legacy lives. This area of the deathbed ecosystem consists of the thoughts your loved one has about their life and what they would like to be remembered for. The topics in this dimension include what brought meaning to your loved one's life, what they think is their most important contribution to the world, how they would like to be remembered, and if there is any wisdom they would like to pass on.

The skills used in this area are similar to the emotional domain. They include talking and listening. Specific tasks that can be performed are working to create a legacy project with your loved one with photos, journals, a digital memory book, or collecting their stories. This area can bring a lot of fun and bonding to the deathbed ecosystem. Once projects are completed, they can be used when your loved one is further in their dying journey by you to connect with them or those around the bedside.

CONNECTION PRACTICE: Recipe Book: Preserving Flavorful Memories

Create a tangible legacy of shared meals and memories.

Purpose: To celebrate your loved one's connection to food and preserve their culinary traditions for future generations.

Time needed: Initial gathering: 1-2 hours; Compilation: 3-4 hours (can be spread over days or weeks)

Instructions:

1. If your loved one has a passion for cooking or a deep connection to food, begin gathering their favorite recipes, whether handwritten, passed down through generations, or from treasured sources.
2. Use this as an opportunity to spark conversation with your loved one and others, reminiscing about the meals and flavors that have shaped their life.
3. Include notes, stories, or special memories that relate to each dish.
4. Compile these into a keepsake book that can be shared with family members.

Reflection: How do these recipes tell the story of your loved one's life? What values and traditions are embedded in these culinary practices?

CONNECTION PRACTICE: Candle Lighting Ceremony

Create a ritual that connects those present with those at a distance.

Purpose: To establish a regular practice that honors your loved one and creates a moment of connection for everyone who cares about them.

Time needed:10-15 minutes weekly

Instructions:

1. Choose a day and time each week to honor your loved one by lighting a candle.
2. This practice can begin while they are still at the bedside, allowing both those present and those unable to be there to participate.
3. As the candle is lit, invite everyone to share something special about your loved one—whether aloud or in quiet reflection.
4. This ritual can continue even after your loved one has passed as a way to keep their memory alive.

Reflection: How does creating a ritual influence your experience of grief? What emerges in these moments of intentional remembrance?

THE SPIRITUAL DOMAIN: FINDING MEANING AND TRANSCENDENCE

The spiritual domain of the dying process is where your loved one or yourself may search for meaning in the experience or the life they lived. This area is often guided by religious or philosophical beliefs, but those are not required. In the deathbed ecosystem, one's spirituality need not be tied to a worldly set of beliefs.

As a dying person, your loved one may experience things that are far beyond your realm of comprehension. They may gain clarity or a different perspective on the events and relationships in their life. Then again, they may not. Openness is essential to attending to this area of the dying process. If your loved one was not a religious or spiritual person in their everyday life, do not pressure them to change their beliefs or attitudes in their dying time. If religion or spirituality was important in their everyday life, help them bring it fully into their dying time.

But know that even people without spiritual beliefs or practices can have thoughts about this part of their dying process. The topics in this dimension include what your loved one believes happens when someone dies, if they would like any religious/nonreligious ceremonies performed before they die, and whether or not they would like support in discussing any existential phenomena.

Tasks that can be performed to meet the needs of this domain include but are not limited to performing cultural/spiritual/religious/ritualistic practices to honor your loved one, such as drumming, singing, reading poems or scripture, reading from favorite books, or even watching their favorite sports team. A person's spiritual life is not limited to practices defined by our society as "spiritual." Instead, think of your loved one's spiritual life as the things in life that made their heart sing. For some, that was a church. For others, that may be listening to public radio or watching their football team. Be open. Your definition of what constitutes a spiritual pursuit may not be in line with what your loved one defines it as. And just like the other domains, you will not know your loved one's thoughts on this area unless you have asked them questions and truly listened to their answers.

WRITING REFLECTION: Contemplating the Afterlife

Create space to explore beliefs about what happens after death.

Purpose: To reflect on personal beliefs about the afterlife, regardless of religious background, which can bring comfort and perspective during this time.

Time needed: 5-10 minutes for writing, with additional time for reflection

Instructions:

1. Take a moment to sit with your thoughts and consider what you believe Heaven or the afterlife looks like.
2. This practice can be meaningful for anyone, regardless of religious background, so feel free to reframe the question to explore what you think happens after death.
3. Begin by writing down your thoughts, allowing your ideas to flow freely onto the page.
4. Once you have finished writing, take a moment to read over what you've written.
5. Sit quietly with the words and allow yourself to feel whatever arises from within.

Reflection: Did anything surprise you about your own beliefs? How might these reflections influence how you approach your loved one's spiritual needs?

THE PRACTICAL DOMAIN: MANAGING LOGISTICS AND PLANNING

The practical domain of the dying process overlaps with the other domains in that it is where the planning discussed in the other areas meets logistics and action. This is also the area where after-death planning comes into play. The practical domain is where arrangements are made for support like home health care, adjusting the physical features of the home, locating a desirable facility if staying at home is not feasible, finding people to shop for groceries, or running errands.

Planning for how your loved one's body will be cared for once they have died, any funeral, or celebration of life arrangements are both parts of this dimension. Topics in this area include where your loved one would like to spend the rest of their life- at home, in a facility, or in a family member's home – and if it is logistically and financially possible. Also included is who will be able to provide care, whether it is professional care or informal, community care, and when that care will take place.

Lastly, this domain reaches into the area of what will happen once your loved one has stopped living. Questions that can be asked to guide decisions in the practical domain include what physical environment would your loved one like to spend their dying time in, who would your loved one like to be in charge of relaying information about their dying journey to people in the community, and what type of event would your loved one like to honor their life?

CONNECTION PRACTICE: Host a Living Funeral

Create a celebration of life while your loved one can participate.

Purpose: To allow your loved one to experience the love, memories, and impact of their life while they are still present to receive it.

Time needed: Planning: Several days to weeks; Event: 2-4 hours (or multiple shorter gatherings)

Instructions:

1. Consider hosting a "living funeral" as a way to celebrate your loved one while they are still present.
2. Begin by selecting a venue for the event, keeping in mind what your loved one enjoys in their daily life.
3. The nature of the event can be as simple or elaborate as you wish—tailored to their preferences and interests.
4. If your loved one is unable to leave their current location, choose a time and day for a group of loved ones to visit them.
5. You may want to spread the celebration over multiple days, depending on the circumstances.
6. Be sure to document the event with photos, videos, and written messages.
7. Provide guests with books where they can write messages or memories.

Reflection: What did this experience reveal about your loved one's impact on others? How did experiencing this celebration influence your loved one's perspective on their life?

BALANCING CARE ACROSS THE DOMAINS

No one person should be made to feel that it is their job to attend to every dimension of their loved one's dying process. Coping theories in psychology state that if the perceived demands of a situation exceed the resources available, then there may be a decrease in the quality of life. It is my hope that you are learning to balance the demands of supporting your loved one during their end-of-life journey while asking for help when you need it.

If you have conversations that define what your loved one's end-of-life wishes are, then identify and mobilize your resources accordingly, then maybe, just maybe, you will not be knocked over so far by your loved one's dying time. That is not to say that what you are going through is not hard. It is. There is no way around that, but maybe through reading this book, you will find the strength to reach out for help when you need it and even before. Managing your energy level and resources when supporting your loved one is like managing pain. It is easier to stay ahead of pain by regularly taking prescribed medications than it is to catch up on pain once it starts. You can better support your loved one if you stay ahead of your own needs and distribute the weight and levels of caregiving across many people.

4

END-OF-LIFE PLANNING

Now, I will provide you with tangible ideas for setting up your loved one's deathbed ecosystem and creating a values-based care plan for their end-of-life journey. By doing this, you will be able to advocate for their needs. A values-based care plan will ensure their comfort, dignity, and preferred quality of life during their final days by incorporating their beliefs, desired location for care, preferred level of medical intervention, and who they want to be involved in decision-making.

End-of-life planning often begins with completing the necessary medical, legal, and financial paperwork. It is the documents and decisions part of end-of-life planning. This part of the book is not meant to substitute legal, financial, or medical advice. It is intended to educate you on the types of documents that might benefit your loved one during their dying time. Please find professionals such as doctors, lawyers, and financial advisors to complete specific paperwork.

The business part of dying is often the easiest and most well-known area for people to address when it comes to end-of-life planning. Although it can still be an intense experience, the practical nature of completing end-of-life documents and working with what is known in life- finances, assets, insurance, utilities, and how to handle them can be a great starting point in end-of-life conversations. This is the part of end-of-life planning that is supported by a legal professional. Depending on the client's situation, a financial professional may also be involved in this part of the planning process. The paperwork that is typically included in this area of the business of dying includes wills and durable and/or financial power of attorney. This is the area where estate planning, life insurance policies, and trusts live. The more complex a living person's financial lifestyle is, the more intricate this area of planning will be. But not every person requires complex forms. It is all dependent upon your loved one's life. The practical part of the medical journey of death should be completed, taking into consideration your loved one's diagnosis and potential needs that relate to that diagnosis and may need input from a physician and/or your loved one's palliative or hospice care team.

This section of the book has questions for you to consider and to ask your loved one. Completing documents and making decisions about end-of-life requires patient and open conversations, which may be difficult for your loved one or yourself. Take your time with this material, and remember, while you may have ideas about what is best for your loved one, it is important to keep in mind they are at the center of these conversations and decisions. Not every question in this book needs to be asked. And not every question will have a clear answer. Think of this work as a starting point to give you the courage to find your own way to engage your loved one in what they would like to see happen during their dying journey.

This is also a time to consider another death doula skill-pacing. What I mean by pacing is that when you ask your loved one questions about end-of-life planning, do not do it in a rapid-fire style. Take your time with them, take a breath, and follow your loved one's lead. Death doulas are trained to mirror the tempo of their clients in terms of breath, energy levels, and conversations.

You may encounter difficulty in this conversation if your loved one is not ready to face the truth of their circumstances. If that happens, know that there may be several reasons behind their unwillingness to talk about their end of life. Give them some space and grace to feel how they do in the moment. Come back later and try to ask a question. By being patient and not forcing questions on your loved one, you show them they have a say in their life when they may feel out of control, disappointed, or betrayed by their body. This builds trust and safety with your loved one. It shows them they still have power and agency in their life, even as it is ending.

You may find that your loved one already has everything planned out. In that case, wonderful! All they need to do is share where the documents are and who is in charge of ensuring their wishes are fulfilled to the best of their abilities. I have known people to say that they have all their affairs in order when what they actually have are ideas in their heads.

One story that comes back to me is about my dear friend Laurie and her mom. After Laurie's dad passed away several years ago, her mom made a big deal about telling her daughter that all of her affairs were in order. All Laurie would have to do when her mom began her end-of-life journey would be to find the folder in the file cabinet. Everything Laurie would need during her mom's dying time was in that folder. Since the reality of the work involved in managing her dad's end-of-life caregiving and funeral planning was fresh in her mind, Laurie decided to peek at her mom's end-of-life wishes folder. For some people, part of the grieving process can involve confirming important people in their lives have communicated end-of-life wishes in legal, binding documents. I did this after my mom died. I needed to know that my dad had his paperwork in order and where it was. Then, I organized my husband's and my personal end-of-life paperwork. It was as though sifting through papers and clarifying our decisions provided a sense of safety and relief during a time when the complexity of my emotions was too much.

Laurie may have felt emotions similar to mine when she peeked into her mom's file cabinet. She may have wanted to better prepare herself for what was to be when her mom started her end-of-life journey one day. What Laurie found in the file was indeed what her mom wanted... what music she wanted to play at her funeral. As you can guess, the information that was lacking in the end-of-life folder existed, but only in Laurie's mom's head. This meant they had to have some gentle conversations about the documents and decisions that would make up Laurie's mom's values-based care plan for end-of-life.

CREATING A VALUES-BASED CARE PLAN: END-OF-LIFE PLANNING

Understanding End-of-Life Documentation: A brief summary of key paperwork to ensure your loved one's wishes are honored.

A well-organized care plan begins with the necessary legal and medical documentation. These documents ensure your loved one's wishes are respected and that those responsible for their care have the clarity and authority to act when needed.

Legal Planning Documents

- Will - Directs how assets should be distributed and names an executor
- Financial Power of Attorney (POA) - Designates someone to handle financial matters
- Trusts - May help avoid probate and manage assets (if applicable)
- Declaration for Disposition of Final Remain-Outlines preferences for body disposition and ceremonial rites

Medical Documents

- Advance Directive – Includes a living will and healthcare proxy designation.
- Medical Power of Attorney (Medical POA) – Appoints someone to make healthcare decisions.
- DNR Order (Do Not Resuscitate) – Instructs providers not to perform CPR
- POLST/MOLST(Physician/Medical Orders for Life-Sustaining Treatment) – Offers specific medical orders for individuals with serious illness

Personal Planning Documents

- Funeral and Burial Instructions – Specifies desired arrangements and services.
- Legacy Letter / Ethical Will – A heartfelt message conveying values, memories, or guidance

- Personal Property Memorandum – Designates specific personal belongings to recipients
- Important Contact Information – Includes professionals, caregivers, and key personal contacts.

Note: The complexity of these documents will depend on your loved one's life circumstances. Not everyone requires elaborate forms or complex arrangements—the key is ensuring that the essentials are covered in a way that reflects their wishes and needs.

Questions to Guide End-of-Life Paperwork Planning

Document Status and Storage

- What documents are already in place? (e.g., Will, POA, Medical POA, Advance Directive, DNR)
- Where are the originals stored?
- Do the named individuals have access to the paperwork?

Decision-Making Roles

- Who is designated as power of attorney and medical power of attorney?
- Would your loved one prefer different people for medical and financial decisions?
- If no one is designated yet, who would they trust in these roles?

Body Disposition

- Is there a Declaration for Disposition of Final Remains form? (This form allows your loved one to make a written declaration, including their wishes as to how they want their body to be disposed of and what ceremonial rites they want to occur after they pass away. Many times in a Last Will and Testament, there will be a clause providing for funeral and burial arrangements).
- What are your loved one's wishes regarding burial, cremation, or ceremonies?

Tips for Managing End-of-Life Documents

- Keep originals in a secure but accessible location (avoid safety deposit boxes that may be difficult to access quickly)
- Provide copies to healthcare providers and ask them to be added to the digital medical record.
- Give copies to the designated POAs and key family members
- Talk to close relatives about these plans to avoid misunderstandings and emotional conflict later on

PAUSE AND REFLECT EXERCISE: Document Inventory

Purpose: To clarify which documents are complete and which still need attention

Time Needed: 30–60 minutes

Instructions:

1. Gather all existing legal and medical documents.
2. Review the guiding questions above.
3. Create an inventory of what documents are present and what's missing.
4. Record where each document is stored.

Reflection: What surprised you about the document inventory process? Were there any unexpected gaps or concerns?

MEDICAL CONSIDERATIONS IN END-OF-LIFE PLANNING

Planning for the medical aspects of end-of-life care helps ensure that care aligns with personal values and comfort preferences. This conversation needs to take into account your loved one's past medical and life experiences. They may be leery of medical professionals such as hospice and palliative care workers. They may want only professionals to provide certain aspects of their care.

Questions to Explore:

- What treatments would your loved one accept or refuse (e.g., feeding tubes, ventilators)?
- Are there specific physical conditions that would make life feel no longer meaningful?
- If a family member wants a treatment your loved one doesn't, how should that be handled?
- Are there physical aspects of dying that cause fear?
- Who would your loved one prefer to provide intimate care (e.g., hygiene)? Is there anyone they'd prefer not to involve?

PAUSE AND REFLECT EXERCISE: **Medical Preferences Discussion**

Purpose: To explore and document your loved one's medical wishes and concerns

Time Needed: 45–60 minutes, with flexibility for breaks

Instructions:

1. Choose a quiet, comfortable space to talk.
2. Go through the medical questions above at a calm pace.
3. Document responses using your loved one's exact words when possible.
4. Revisit this conversation periodically, as preferences may evolve.

Reflection: What insights emerged from this discussion? Were there any emotional moments, fears, or values that stood out?

Location of Care: Home vs. Facility

Many people say that they want to die at home, but it is often not able to happen because of a lack of proper planning, financial resources, or not enough physical support. The decision between dying at home and in a facility is not one that many people make. Without prior talks about the topic of where your loved one would like to spend their dying time, they will often end up wherever their situation takes them.

Factors to Consider:

- Medical needs and whether they can be met at home
- Availability and capacity of family caregivers
- Financial resources for home care support
- Suitability of the home for care (e.g., accessibility)
- Proximity to medical services
- Local hospice resources (in-home and facility-based)

Note: Without prior planning, individuals may end up in a care setting that wasn't their preference. Discussing this early can make all the difference.

Medication Management

Your loved one may have many medications that need to be given at various times over the day. If hospice is being used, then they should instruct caregivers on how and when to administer medications. It is helpful to have a medication log sheet where information is collected on when and how much of a medication was given. If no medication log is provided to you, do an online search for free medication logs to print out. You can always use a spreadsheet, too. Use whatever makes this part of caregiving easiest for those providing care.

Tips for Medication Management:

- Use a medication log to track dosage times and amounts
- Set alarms or reminders for medication times
- Utilize a spreadsheet, printable log, or medication app
- Keep a master list of medications, purposes, and potential side effects
- Designate a lead caregiver to oversee medication responsibilities

Creating the Complete Care Plan

A comprehensive values-based care plan integrates all these elements—legal documents, medical preferences, location choices, and practical considerations—into a cohesive guide that honors your loved one's wishes while providing clear direction for caregivers.

Remember that this plan may need to evolve as your loved one's condition changes. Regular check-ins about preferences and needs will help ensure the plan remains aligned with their wishes as their journey unfolds.

By approaching end-of-life planning thoughtfully and comprehensively, you create a foundation that supports not just the practical aspects of care but the emotional, spiritual, and relational dimensions as well—allowing everyone involved to focus on what matters most during this precious time.

5

CREATING SACRED SPACE

The idea that a dying person could still have quality in their life may be irritating, foreign, or ridiculous sounding, but it is true. Everyone's definition of quality of life is unique, and it changes based on their current physical, mental, and spiritual states.

I had the privilege of attending the bedside of a family friend, Tom. Tom's terminal diagnosis and progression through the dying process were speedy. I did not spend much time at his bedside, but during the time I did, I realized his transition was my ideal scenario for what a sacred dying space could be.

TOM'S SACRED SPACE: A MODEL OF END-OF-LIFE CARE

When I walked into the house, I was greeted immediately with the sounds of family members of all ages moving about. The front office in the home had been reallocated to Tom's bedroom. In it, he lay on a hospital bed surrounded by various chairs. Bedside tables were close by to set the supplies, such as mouth swabs used to aid his dry mouth and washcloths to wipe his face on. Boxes of tissues were placed throughout the space. His oxygen concentrator was sitting outside his room to reduce ambient noises.

There were people everywhere- some were community members coming for a visit, others were family members chatting with each other or with Tom. The kitchen was full of food needed to sustain those doing the fulfilling and taxing work of caregiving.

The entire house was focused on supporting Tom while still allowing those who lived there to attend to their daily tasks. Tom's grandkids ran about the house- playing, doing homework, and coming in to sit calmly on their grandfather's bed.

His wife, Connie, was his primary caregiver, along with her two children. They also had a hospice team that brought medical supplies and came to check on the family daily. This was not Connie's first time caregiving for a loved one at the end of life. Connie was also a nurse, so she understood what Tom's body was doing. She could easily explain the physical aspects of what was happening to her kids and grandkids.

When Tom entered the hospital and received his terminal diagnosis, he told Connie he wanted to go home. She listened. Through the times that they had supported other members of their family through the dying process, Tom and Connie had talked about and learned what was important to them for their own end-of-life journeys.

THE RELIEF OF UNDERSTANDING

I clearly remember the look on Connie's face when I showed up in Tom's room. Her shoulders dropped, and she hugged me. It was as though this strong, capable woman was holding it all together for her husband, her family, and their social circle. Nurses are trained to do that- put the needs of others before their own.

When I walked into the space as a person trained in deathcare, comfortable with all the dimensions of dying, Connie relaxed. I had no expectation that Tom would survive, which relieved any pressure she may have felt. I confirmed that Tom looked good and was well cared for, being surrounded by so much life and love.

I had to explain to someone what I meant by "good" because they did not equate the idea that someone could look good and be dying. As a deathcare and former healthcare professional, I understand what the body does as a person dies. When I said "good," I meant that Tom was progressing as he should in the dying process, and he looked comfortable and well-cared for. He did not show signs of pain or distress. My words were not spoken to give the impression that he would recover.

QUALITY IN THE FINAL DAYS

Although Tom's diagnosis was unexpected and his disease progressed quickly, he was able to make decisions about where and how he wanted to spend his last days. His quality of life was good. Just like in daily living, when people are dying, they have good days and bad ones. The baseline of what good and bad means for an individual shifts based on where they are in the dying process.

Tom was no longer mobile or speaking. He was still able to take small amounts of liquids and occasionally give a hand squeeze. He was never going to get up and ride his bicycle around town or work again, but he was able to have a few drops of his favorite beer, which had been okay with his hospice nurse.

Tom died quietly at home, surrounded by his family. No

one wanted him to get sick or die, but everyone could see that his body was no longer able to hold him here.

THE NATURAL PROGRESSION

A dying person moves through their dying time by letting go of their physical body. Sometimes, this process is quick, like my mom's dying time. Other times, it takes longer, like in Robert's case. Hopefully, it can be accomplished with little suffering. Just like being born, the labor of death moves on its own timeline.

CREATING YOUR LOVED ONE'S SACRED SPACE

Supporting a loved one through their final days involves thoughtful preparation of their physical and emotional environment. This section offers questions and guidance to help create a peaceful, supportive, and sacred space aligned with your loved one's needs and preferences.

Guiding Questions for Setting Up a Sacred Space

Location of Care

- Where does your loved one want to be cared for? (e.g., home, hospice facility, nursing facility, family member's home)
- Is dying at home physically and financially feasible?

Home Environment Assessment

- Does the home provide enough space for necessary equipment?

- Is there a room large enough to serve as a care space?
- Are doorways wide enough for wheelchairs or furniture?
- Is there a bathroom nearby?
- Is there space for the primary caregiver to rest?

Daily Routines and Emotional Comfort

- What are your loved one's important routines or rituals?
- Which activities bring them joy or comfort?
- How can these routines be preserved—or new ones created—to maintain dignity and familiarity?

Communication and Preferences

- What is your loved one's desired level of information sharing about their condition?
- Where do they feel most comfortable?
- Are there physical discomforts (e.g., smell, noise, lighting, fabric, touch) that should be avoided?
- What kind of music, sounds, or silence do they prefer?
- Are there comfort items like a favorite blanket, chair, or temperature setting?
- Do they want pets nearby for companionship?

Tips for Setting Up the Space

If at Home:

- Choose a quiet room, ideally on the main level, with natural light and space for caregivers and equipment.
- Keep the space tidy but welcoming, allowing room for visitors and professionals.
- A hospital bed can improve comfort and adjustability.
- Have extra pillows for propping and positioning.
- Use cups with straws or droppers to offer liquids. Do not give liquids to someone who is unconscious.
- Use mouth swabs or a damp washcloth to moisten lips; lip balm can soothe dryness.
- Keep linens and supplies close to reduce caregiver burden.
- Dispose of absorbent products like adult briefs and absorbent pads outside to reduce odor.

Hospice staff will supply many medical supplies like adult briefs and absorbent pads. If you are not using hospice, then order supplies from Amazon or another home delivery service to save time. This can also be an area where caregivers make lists of supplies needing to be picked up for people who offer help.

If in a Facility:

- Personalize the room with familiar items to create a home-like environment.

Enhancing Comfort Through the Five Senses

No matter where your loved one ends up spending the remainder of their life, you can make their space a little more comfortable by focusing on the five senses when choosing what elements to bring into their deathbed ecosystem. This is easier to do at home, but do not be afraid to bring items that create a homelike environment for your loved one into a facility. All of these ideas are offerings. Use them as they best serve your loved one and yourself. With many of them, gaining your loved one's consent is important, especially with touch.

Sight

- Place framed photos of loved ones and meaningful moments around the room.
- Position the bed near a window with a view.
- Bring in photo albums or memory boards.
- Display artwork made by children or family members.

Sound

- Play favorite music or soothing background playlists using a speaker or phone.
- Use white noise machines to block disruptive sounds in shared facilities.
- Consider live music, music therapy, or simple singing.

Touch

- Cover your loved one with a favorite blanket or quilt.
- Choose clothing that is soft, non-restrictive, and easy to change (e.g., back-slit shirts).
- Offer gentle hand or foot massages with alcohol-free lotion.
- Hold their hand, with permission.

Taste

- Keep favorite snacks and beverages on hand if they can eat or drink safely.
- Offer small, easy-to-eat meals.
- Use taste and smell together to comfort even when full meals aren't possible.

Smell

- Keep fresh flowers or fragrant plants nearby.
- Use diffusers or lightly spray familiar perfumes on pillows.
- Allow fresh air to circulate, or use an air purifier to maintain freshness.

Social Considerations

Lastly, when setting up your loved one's deathbed ecosystem, consider their social baseline prior to their dying process. People who were private prior to starting the dying process may remain private. They may not want many people at their bedside, or at least they may not want very many visitors all at once. Social people may be okay with more people visiting at the same time. They may want more of a party environment at times. Your loved one could also swing from being social one day to being private another. As your loved one moves further into their dying process, they may become less interested in the world outside of themselves. Use your best judgment as to how many people can visit and how long they can visit when your loved one enters this stage of their dying process.

PART III

BEING PRESENT

6

THE ART OF PRESENCE

The word presence is defined in the Merriam-Webster dictionary as "the fact or condition of being present." Thanks, dictionary. Your description is not very helpful when applied to thinking about how to best be with a loved one in their dying time. Looking up the word "present" yields definitions of "aiming, pointing, or directing something in a particular direction, making a gift to someone, or being in view." All of these definitions provide a logical understanding of the word, *and* they all lack depth in explaining the act of being present with someone, especially someone who knows that they are dying.

Doug Silsbee, the founder of Presence-Based Coaching, said that presence is a "devilishly slippery and challenging word to define." Doug died in 2018 from cancer. For much of his career, Doug focused on teaching others to live in the present, and he continued to do so after his diagnosis and in his dying time. He defined presence as a state of being, not a verb, noun, or adjective. It is an "in the moment" awareness characterized by connectedness to others and to self. Presence creates a feeling of timelessness that can open people up to the larger truths of the world by developing an expansiveness within oneself. This allows us to see clearly and directly who people are, their situations, and how everyone fits into a bigger picture together. I again agree with Mr. Silsbee. Presence is bigger and deeper than simple words can describe. It is expansive, and it allows you to connect with yourself and your loved one in surprising ways.

It may seem as though presence is something that has to be taught and mastered when, in fact, it already exists within you. Being present does not require extensive training, expensive degrees, credentials, or years of experience. All it asks of you is self-awareness, compassion, and practice. It does not have a high price tag, nor does it ask you to be perfect.

Why is it important for you to practice in the time you have left with your loved one? Because presence is a gift. It is one of the most powerful and simple ways to show love, respect, and support during someone's dying time. It creates a human-to-human connection with your loved one without struggling to fix an unwanted circumstance. Presence affirms your loved one's personhood and autonomy at a time when they may not feel valued or like they belong here anymore. It offers quiet security and comfort in silence. Practicing presence nourishes both of your souls while you face your current reality so that you may be better equipped to face your future.

Before I go on and on about the benefits of practicing presence, I must acknowledge that our current world has us trained to disengage from ourselves and those around us. We turn to easy distractions like our phones, food, junk television, alcohol, and many other indulgences that we overuse to get by in our daily lives. Add in the difficult situation you are facing, the act of being present may be even harder for you.

Let me take this moment to express that distractions are

sometimes necessary for you as you act as a companion for your loved one. This is not an easy road for you to travel. It is even tougher for them. So remember to be gentle with your expectations of yourself and everyone else who shows up at the bedside. Give yourself a break occasionally. And as with every section of this book, my ideas are an invitation for you to consider something. My words are not commands or declarations of the right way to support your dying person. It is always within your power to choose whether something I offer is right for your loved one and you. So, with that, let's get into the practical aspects of practicing presence.

THE BENEFITS OF PRACTICING PRESENCE

The benefits of practicing presence at the bedside include cultivating and maintaining love between the people surrounding your loved one. It also aids in making stressful events less challenging by providing you with a way to relax while helping you accept the reality of the moment. Presence helps you find comfort in natural silences. This practice can also establish your ability to recognize and manage emotions.

The human-to-human connection created with presence begins first with a self-to-self connection. What I mean by this is that you have to open yourself up and notice first what is going on inside of you before you can truly be with another person. This takes being vulnerable, which can be especially challenging when accompanying someone at the end of their life because there can be so many unknowns in the journey. Plus, the vastness of your emotions and any relationship entanglements you may have with your loved one can affect your physical body, your thinking self, and your emotional self. However, vulnerability is a starting point for belonging, and when you feel at home with yourself, your ability to feel at home with others increases. That grounded, at-home feeling is a basis for walking fully into the presence of another person.

JOCELYN'S STORY: TAKING TIME AND SPACE

Jocelyn received my help with her grandfather's end-of-life journey after growing tired of not having anyone willing to listen to her struggles with watching this man become weak. Our work together was not planned. We began talking about Jocelyn's situation at a community event. She shared with an acquaintance that she chose to spend time with family instead of attending the last gathering. I was not a part of this conversation, but something made my ears catch what the acquaintance asked her next… She asked Jocelyn if she was close to her grandfather and how old he was. She then told Jocelyn that it is not so hard to lose a family member when they are old and the relationship is not a close one like a grandparent-grandchild relationship. At that point, I turned towards Jocelyn and waited until the other lady moved on to another conversation. I could see how the acquaintance's words impacted Jocelyn. She was struggling to make her internal world match what her friend had just told her that her reality should be. She should not be upset over what her elderly grandpa was going through. He lived a long life, and he had not been very involved with her during her childhood. It was then that I placed a hand gently on her forearm and said, "It is okay to be upset when someone you know is dying. It doesn't matter if they are old and have lived a long life; it can still hurt to see them die. It doesn't even matter if you have a close relationship. Give yourself time and space to feel what you feel about your grandfather." Jocelyn placed her hand on top of mine and said, "Thank you. I needed to hear that."

Our short exchange led to our working together during

the rest of her grandpa's dying time. By working, I mean quick texts, in-person conversations, or a few minutes of shared silence where she could let down her guard because she knew I was okay with her showing up just how she was. I did not tell her how she should feel about anything. I allowed her to be cracked open and vulnerable as we stood in the presence of her experience.

In our conversations, Jocelyn and I worked on ways for her to connect with her feelings, thoughts, and emotions without feeling overwhelmed. We did this by having her practice a quick and simple self-witnessing exercise. This practice is adapted from Manuela Mischke-Reeds, MA, LMFT. The intention of this exercise is to create space in your internal environment to train yourself to take pauses. Practicing pauses, especially when acting as a companion for a loved one in their dying journey, brings an expansiveness to your awareness, which sets the stage for presence.

COPING EXERCISE: Self-Witness Practice

Create a moment of present awareness to ground yourself during stressful times.

Purpose: To interrupt automatic patterns of stress and reconnect with your sensory experience, creating a reset point during challenging moments.

Time needed: 1-3 minutes

Instructions:

1. Suspend: Hit the pause button on anything that you are doing.
2. Notice: Observe your environment with attention to each sense:
3. Don't Judge: Track what you observe without judgment. In this moment, there is no good, no bad. There just is.
   - What do you hear in your environment?
   - What do you see in the space around you?
   - Do you smell anything or taste anything?
   - What sensations are present in your physical body?
4. Breathe deeply: Take several conscious breaths before returning to what you were doing.

Reflection: How does this brief pause change your relationship to what you were doing? What shifts in your body, emotions, or thoughts after this simple practice?

~

One item that I teach my clients is the concept of Me- She-We. Feel free to insert whatever pronouns work for you into this idea. I have a fitness instructor who likes to say, "Control your body, and you will control your life." This concept is problematic for me because I believe that I (the "me" -my thoughts, my emotions, and my stories) work in concert with my body (the "she"- my felt senses and my body's abilities) to create a "we" which is the combined awareness of all types of intelligence. I believe we have intelligence, or knowing, in all areas of our being, not just our minds. This idea is based on works from Wilhelm Reich, Bessel van der Kolk, Peter

Levin, and many others, in addition to my observations of others and myself as we deal with somatic or body sensations during stressful situations. As humans, if we spend too much time or energy controlling one aspect of the me-she-we dynamic, then our innate intelligence will speak up. An example of this in my life is when I take on too much responsibility, and my lumbar spine tries to take me out by becoming unstable and painful. My being knows I am stressed and wants me to take a break. If I do not listen to my needs, my back provides a reason for me to rest. Another example of how our being's various intelligences work to inform us is how a client of mine becomes thirsty when we discuss her unexpressed wants and needs. It is almost as though her being was parched after her unmet needs and wants were expressed, which turned into thirst or a cry out for more. The conversation around my client's physical reaction to the topic helped her connect to herself and gave her a way to listen to the signal her being was providing her.

So let's bring this idea of me-she-we back to you and see if you can begin to listen to what your being is telling you as you support your loved one during their dying time. This practice is an invitation to work on your self-to-self connection and awareness. Answering the following questions is not a requirement. You can skip over them and come back to them later if thinking about them is too difficult, or you can choose to not read them at all.

PAUSE AND REFLECT EXERCISE: Me-She-We Practice

Explore your emotional patterns and interactions during your caregiving journey.

Purpose: To develop an awareness of your response patterns in different situations, helping you navigate the emotional complexity of end-of-life caregiving with greater self-understanding.

Time needed: 15-20 minutes in a quiet, private setting

Instructions:

1. Reflect on Pleasant Moments
   - Think about a recent pleasant situation. How did you feel emotionally?
   - Notice how your body responded. Were you relaxed? Energized? At ease?
   - Consider interactions with others during this time. What did they say or do? How did they respond to you?
   - How do you typically celebrate or savor these moments of joy or peace?
2. Reflect on Mildly Stressful Moments
   - Shift your attention to moments that were mildly or moderately stressful (not overwhelming).
   - Take a deep breath and notice how your body reacts to stressful situations.
   - What emotions typically arise? Do you become emotionally or physically needy?

   - How did others perceive you during these times? What feedback did they offer?
   - Note any patterns in your physical responses to stress.
3. Bring Yourself to the Present Moment
   - Gently shift your focus to your current experience with your loved one's end-of-life journey.
   - Notice any physical sensations that arise when you think about this experience.
   - Reflect on how others are interacting with you during this time.
   - Are you over-functioning (taking on too many responsibilities) or under-functioning (feeling emotionally drained)?
   - What emotions are present? Note them without judgment.
4. Integrating Insights
   - Consider how these insights can inform how you respond to your loved one's journey.
   - Identify emotional or physical patterns you might want to adjust.
   - Reflect on how you can better support your own needs throughout this process.
   - Consider how to create space for your emotions while maintaining balance.

Reflection: What patterns did you notice across different situations? How might awareness of these patterns help you navigate challenging moments in your caregiving journey? What one small change could you make based on these insights?

Taking time to answer questions like these can help deepen your awareness of your experience, which allows you to notice others' experiences. Remember, acknowledging intense emotions or body sensations that come up takes courage. It should not push you over the edge of no return. If it does feel like it's too much to give your felt sense and emotional being space to be recognized, then stop. Back off and acknowledge less intense sensations or feelings like how cold you get while sitting at your loved one's medical appointments or how you enjoy the way the sky looks out the window.

Giving yourself time to feel what you are feeling does not have to take long or start with deep thoughts to be effective. A few seconds here and there may help, even if what you are noticing is trivial in comparison to the bigger situation at hand. Developing an ease with noticing, acknowledging, and sharing your felt sense, thoughts, and emotions takes practice. You can always come back to it. Although, if at any moment your situation feels like it is unmanageable for you, then seek help from a social worker, a chaplain, a therapist, a friend, a family member, or even your physician. Asking for help can be hard, but it does not mean there is anything wrong with you.

Humans are communal creatures in life and in death. Witnessing all that is involved with another human approaching the end of life is big work. Give yourself permission to be vulnerable- ask for help when you need it, take a break when you can, and connect with yourself and your experience.

Feeling overwhelmed may mean it is time to engage in a healthy distraction or that you need to connect with someone outside of the dying space. Remember, by choosing to be present for your loved one during their dying time, you are choosing to be courageous. As Brene Brown says, "There is no courage without vulnerability. Courage requires the willingness to lean into uncertainty, risk, and emotional exposure." Her words were not meant to describe what it is like to accompany another human to the end of their life, but I can't help but think they do anyway.

When you come together in the dying space of your loved one, the interactions of all attending join together to create one interaction. It is a magical thing to witness while also being quietly heartbreaking. Engaging in being present can aid the joining by creating a beautiful energy that surrounds and holds your dying loved one. When you can create a self-to-self connection as you accompany your loved one to the end of their life, you give everyone at the bedside a tremendous gift of your grounding presence.

In my experience at the bedside, it only takes one person bringing that gift to help every person at the moment by creating a safe space that allows all access to their own wisdom to lay the seeds to heal and recover after your loved one leaves their physical body.

COPING EXERCISE: Practicing Presence

Develop the skill of being fully present through mindful seeing.

Purpose: To create a state of non-reactive, nonjudgmental awareness that allows you to be genuinely present with your loved one, even when they cannot fully reciprocate.

Time needed: 5-7 minutes

Instructions:

1. Start by tuning into the awareness of your vision. What do you notice?
2. Focus your eyes on an object in your environment.
3. Allow your eyes to relax and establish a soft-focused view that widens what you see. Tap into your peripheral vision in a way that slightly blurs what is directly in your line of sight.
4. Close your eyes to rest them and allow them to relax. Now, just breathe.
5. Open your eyes without focusing on anything. Soften your gaze and try not to aim your vision at anything.
6. Notice your breathing as you soften your eye sockets.
7. Continue until you feel a relaxation, an ease, or a letting go of your being.
8. Slowly orient your eyes around the room, looking gently while maintaining a soft focus.

Reflection: How does this way of seeing change your experience of your surroundings? What shifts in your body or emotional state when you practice this expansive gaze? How might this presence practice support your interactions with your loved one?

Note: You do not have to maintain this way of seeing indefinitely. With practice, your body will learn to fall into the state of presence using an expansive eye gaze with little effort. When in presence, you see the person in front of you while also opening yourself to be seen, which humanizes all involved.

The keys to presence include self-awareness, a willingness to be vulnerable, an open mindset, and an expansive eye gaze. It is the practice of being present with another even when that person is not fully able to be present with you. It occurs without an agenda or even words. Presence creates a temporary state of non-reactive, nonjudgmental, centered awareness. We have many ways of viewing the world, and often, the way we look out of our eyes is very harsh. How do your eyes feel and look when you are angry? What visual comes to mind when you read someone was seeing with soft eyes, smiling eyes, or teary eyes? Think about how your vision closes in on the screen and its contents when you are looking at your phone while losing connection with the world around you. The ways we see the world with our eyes impact our presence in the world.

7

THE LANGUAGE OF DYING

I was standing at the edge of the table waiting for the customers to give me their order when one of them asked if I was Janet's granddaughter. I said yes. It was not uncommon for the customers at the restaurant to question who I was related to in an attempt to place me on their mental map of people in the town... who were my grandparents, my parents, etc.... This often led people to tell me how they knew my family members or how they were distantly related or connected to me. Except this time, the woman said, "Your grandpa is in a better place. He is with your aunt Micki where he wanted to be." Turns out the woman at the table was friends with my grandmother and knew about the recent hardships in our family. My aunt Micki died at 50 from leukemia after a two-year battle with the disease, and my grandfather died shortly thereafter from prostate cancer. I wasn't expecting her words, and although her sentiment was kind, her statement enraged me. It was too soon after their deaths; it was too unfair that they both got sick, and it hurt too much. I think this was the first time I was consciously aware of the limit words have in describing the experience of losing people I loved.

In retrospect, I know now that my grandmother's friend was trying to express kindness to me while informing her lunch companion about my connection to the family loss. I also remember how this same woman would gingerly ask me about my aunt's health after my aunt's diagnosis when the woman came into the restaurant. She offered no kind words when I would report on my aunt's status.

"Oh, Aunt Micki is finishing up this round of chemo..."

"She is going to move back into Grandma and Grandpa's house after she gets released from the hospital..."

"She is in remission and can move home..."

"The leukemia is back, and she needs a bone marrow transplant..."

"My dad said that I can't go to the hospital to visit anymore because he doesn't want me to remember her like this..."

She never responded with words of wisdom or hard-lived truths. She was my grandmother's age, so I knew she had experienced loss at some point in her life. In fact, I knew her husband had died a few years prior. But she was doing the best she could by asking after my aunt, then responding with a nodding head and a facial expression that matched the information I relayed. I wanted more, though. I wanted words that matched the intensity of the experience of watching a once strong, vibrant loved one become frail and eventually tell her family that she could fight no more. My aunt wanted to die. Continuing treatment was a hopeless cause in her mind, and it was exhausting her. I wanted someone to come along and say something, to give me some kind of label for the situation my family and I were going through because words give credibility to feelings and experiences we have. Somehow, I knew if there was a phrase to describe the journey we had been on with my aunt, then somewhere, another person could relate and see my pain without me even having to speak.

THE LIMITATIONS OF OUR LANGUAGE

Throughout my life and in my work as a death doula, I have learned that there is a limitation in language when it comes to expressing all that takes place when a loved one is dying. What I witnessed in my time as a healthcare worker is we have words in the medical community for when someone is diagnosed with a life-limiting illness or when managing a chronic condition becomes untenable. Oftentimes, those words are focused on fixing or managing the medical aspects of the situation while leaving out the human side. In a world away from healthcare, people offer soft condolences and acts of support. What is missing is that even when we know a person is going to die, that they are terminal, there is no adequate language to describe the place we are all in emotionally, socially, physically, mentally, and spiritually. There are no words that begin to touch the phase between learning that your loved one is going to die and them actively dying. So it is no wonder that we as a culture have little to offer to support people who find themselves in this place in life. We have language to describe role changes after someone dies. A spouse becomes a widow, a child becomes an orphan, but what do you become before your loved one dies, when your time is spent worrying over what is yet to come while you usher them to appointments that all lead to the bedside of their dying time?

In linguistics or the scientific study of language, there is a theory that the language we speak impacts how we view the world. It's called linguistic relativity or sometimes the Sapir-Whorf hypothesis. If this hypothesis is true and we hold the idea that language is the product of a culture, then we can begin to connect how our lack of language around the dying process, especially the early parts before active dying, limits our ability to support the person who is dying and those who surround them because we have no understanding of this phase of life.

HOW OUR PAST SHAPES OUR WORDS

Take a moment and think back on your life and experiences with death and dying. How were they handled? How did the people around you talk about the person who was dying? Was there any talk about family member's feelings throughout the experience? Or was the subject of your loved one's death avoided? Maybe your experience was like mine, and your family and friends did not hide the subject of aging, illness, and dying from the conversation. Maybe, like me, the exposure to these topics allowed you to be better prepared when faced with these life events. Maybe also, like me, when I was forbidden to visit my aunt, there came a point in time when those around you controlled your exposure to the dying process.

Everyone's life is unique, but it is my belief that the way we look at the world is influenced by the way we and the people around us speak or choose not to speak about it. How we show up in our loved one's dying time is shaped by a lifetime of exposure, or lack of it, to death and dying. We, as individuals, are made up of all the people who came before us, what they said, and how they said it. How we support those important to us at their end of life is also influenced by what people around us have said or not said during other's dying times.

LIVING IN THE IN-BETWEEN

Much of my career has been focused on finding language and sentiments to describe the journey to the end of our lives, from the time we receive the news to the active dying process. Because honestly, we are all on a journey to the end of our lives. It is the natural way of the human life cycle. The only thing that separates us is our everyday awareness of our proximity to death. In my time spent looking for words other than terminally ill to describe the person who is dying and for you other than caregiver or family member, I realized that the language to describe the place you both are is limited. I have found many words that fit the experience of getting diagnosed or told that one's life is limited. I have also found many words for the time after someone dies but little for the time in between. The best way I have come up with to describe this place of being is that you inhabit the time between being told that a loved one has something that will end their life and the beginning of the stages of their active dying is still considered living. You are all just living, albeit living in a way that no one wanted. You are in a place of limbo that is difficult to describe to people who have not experienced it and to those who wish not to be reminded of it. Even your loved one who is dying is still living and will continue to do so up until their last breath.

FINDING GRACE IN DIFFICULT CONVERSATIONS

So what does this talk about language mean for someone looking to support a loved one at the bedside during their end-of-life journey? First, it is good to acknowledge that when a loved one is dying, that person and everyone surrounding them hear many words that they never wanted to hear. Language has the power to create a new reality like the one you are living in now. Second, it is good to consider that there is not a correct way to speak about this process. What words comfort one person may cause another upset and that is okay. No one is standing by you with a clipboard, grading your effort to support your loved one, and if they are, then we need to have a different conversation. Seriously, for your loved one, whether a friend or a family member, if your relationship is solid or complicated, your choosing to show up at the bedside for them is a gift. It is a gift for them. It is a gift for you, and gifts are not always easy to give or receive, so give yourself permission to acknowledge how hard all of this is.

Conversations often stop when the topic of death is brought up. It can be a hard subject for many people. It is often avoided, which can make it incredibly hard when a loved one has been told they are dying. Hard for you because few people want a report on the depth of the truth of how it is when a loved one is dying. Hard for your loved one because they are faced with the reality of what used to only happen to others- dying.

Let's be real. There may be a time in everyone's life when they learn a person connected to them is dying, and they don't want to talk about it. That's normal. It is also normal to talk about it. It is my belief that the words we use when talking about death and the timing of when we use them correlate with not only our beliefs around the topic but also where we are in processing and accepting the experience. People who close down when talking about death and dying do so for a reason. It is not our job to find that reason. Being willing to allow those people the space of their discomfort with the experience may open them up. They may feel less pressure and fear when interacting with the person who is dying which could lead to an increase in the connection between them. It is not only the words we speak that have the power to change how we perceive a loved one's dying time, but it is also the pauses between the words that allow everyone present time to catch up with what is taking place.

WHEN WORDS FAIL US

The day my mother died, I experienced how another person's comfort level with death influenced our conversation. The call from my mom's caretaker at 2am that day in May set in motion my challenging process to make it to Indiana before she died. I look back now on the story of my mother's last day alive and see the comfort levels of the different people that I encountered. The airline ticketing agent dug through her computer records to find my ticket when it did not show up in the system after I laid my head on the counter and quietly said, "I need to get home to my dying mom." The people in the security line did not question when a friend much farther in the line noticed me and called me up to her. The irritated stares turned into head turns away or soft glances toward me when I responded to her inquiry about where I was heading. "Home," I said. "My mother is dying today." Then I boarded the plane, taking the last seat by the window in the last row of the plane- not uttering a word during the entire flight, while the two other passengers in my row chatted the entire flight. It wasn't until we started our descent that the lady next to me questioned what she was seeing out the window when I spoke up. She took that as a cue to ask why I was traveling to Indianapolis and how I knew what random buildings were from the air. I told her simply that I was from Indiana and that I was heading home in hopes of seeing my mom one last time before she died. This quieted her. It wasn't until we stood up to exit the plane that she hugged me and told me that she was sure that surely my mom would be okay. I told her no, that there was no way my mom was not dying that day. What I did not know at the time was that my mom had died when I was still in the air and that this stranger was right in a way. My mom was okay. She died a good death, with support from a medical team when she became afraid, my sister, her caretaker, and her brothers at her side. Maybe my seatmate's words were spoken from a place of being fearful of death, that surely modern medicine would save this stranger that she was learning about. Maybe her words were spoken from a place of comfort that if a daughter would fight so hard to make it to a mother's bedside in her last hours, then it was possible that her death would not be so bad. The words shared in that experience have not changed over the years. What has changed is me.

Looking back on the moment with the lady next to me on the plane and comparing how I received her words then to today, I can begin to see examples in my own life of how language- what we say and how we perceive what others say- can relate to where we are at in our personal journey of processing and accepting our loved one's death. That day in 2013, I was not in a place to fully process what was happening. I was in high-function mode. My main thoughts were on supporting my mom and our family. The pauses between the phone calls I made to my sister and my uncles allowed me a little time to reflect, but not much. I had not yet taken enough time to process the range of emotions I was feeling. My mind was managing everything, working hard to protect my heart from the reality of what was happening. It has been over ten years since my mother died, and I think my brain has had enough time to process my grief logically, which gave my heart time to catch up with the loss.

My story shows how our relationship to the death of a loved one can change and how our language around the experience changes, too. Mary Frances O'Conner, PhD, says,

"Grief is a moment that reoccurs over and over." The hole that is created when someone we care about dies does not heal. How we move with it does. I still feel heartbroken over my mom's death, but I speak about it much differently.

DIRECT LANGUAGE VS. GENTLE EUPHEMISMS

It is not unusual for someone trained as a death doula to have a level of comfort with using words like "death" or "dying" instead of things like "passed," "lost," or "gone home." Deathcare workers and the death-positive movement make a point to use direct, clear language to encourage open conversations about the end of life. Unlike the death-positive movement, substitute words or euphemisms for death are often used because it is thought that it will decrease the amount of hurt or shock felt. Plus, it is what we have been taught to say when talking about death. Using words such as "lost" instead of "died" can be confusing to our brain. Researchers say that when we say "lost," our brains assume our loved one can be found somewhere, and that can be unhelpful in processing grief. These softer words might make the healing process easier. Direct and unambiguous words can feel blunt and uncomfortable if the receiver is not ready for them. Substitute phrases create distance from the reality of the event. But, in a way, they can protect both the speaker and receiver because we speak and hear words not just as they are but also as we are. Every thought, every conversation, every look, everything is filtered through the lens of what you have experienced in your life and what you are feeling as your loved one negotiates their dying journey.

As a death doula, it is not my job to walk into a room where someone is dying and correct the words people are using. It is my job to observe, listen, and respond accordingly to everyone present in the space. By inquiring about how best to support your loved one through the entirety of their dying time, you are, in a way, agreeing to do the same. Understanding that people speak and listen based on more than just their thoughts will aid you in connecting with your dying loved one and everyone else present at the bedside. Give people grace when it comes to how they speak about your loved one's dying. Give yourself grace. By gently and slowly bringing in more direct language about the dying process, you will allow people time to soften themselves in a way that brings acceptance of the truth.

8

ALLOWING AND ACCEPTING

There is a special type of patience necessary to allow people you are in a relationship with to follow their inner authority when making choices for themselves. It requires even more patience when the person you are in a relationship with is at the end of their life or dying. It is hard to let go of someone you love. It can even be hard to let go of someone with whom you have had a challenging relationship. Sometimes, those two things exist within the same relationship. There is a complexity of emotions that come up at the end of someone's life- love, sadness, regret, frustration, anger, confusion, guilt... These emotions can lead your loved ones to make certain decisions that you don't agree with. The same goes for the decisions you may make if you are in charge of your loved one if they become incapacitated.

What this means is you could overlook getting input from the person in the bed. While this is a well-intentioned act, it disregards your loved one's autonomy or their sense of ownership of their life and experience. This may especially be true once your loved one reaches a stage in their dying journey where they interact little with those around them.

You may make decisions based on your desire to protect them, to keep them alive for longer than they would like, or agree to treatments that are temporary fixes for an unfixable situation when they want none of it. Or maybe you are operating based on their wishes. Good. Keep it up. Either way- if they share their end-of-life wishes with you in a clear way that can be followed by their family, support professionals, and their community, or if you are making it up as you go, it can be hard to allow your loved one to die.

There is a lot of letting go that has to happen in order to be in a good place with your loved one dying. Maybe saying "a good place" is not the right language, because are you ever really in a good place to live without your loved one? It helps if you can work at letting go of or at least acknowledging expectations, past hurts, fears of the unknown, uncommunicated feelings, judgments, loss of a future together, and so on.

Remember the part of the relational tapestry chapter where I talked about the man in the hospital whose family was not ready to accept that he was at the end of his life? Well, that man was my dad, and I was there not only as a daughter but also as an end-of-life professional.

My dad, with his fragile health, had yet again had another diabetic crisis that landed him in the ICU, teetering on the brink of death. I rushed to town because, over the years, I have learned that every medical crisis could be his last, and I never know if the hospital staff will get him back. Because of the long history he has with mismanaging his health, my sister and I decided enough was enough. It was time for some lifestyle changes for my dad, and by lifestyle, I meant moving into a facility that could monitor his health so the last part of his life could be lived in a higher quality than it currently was. We were not looking to fix him or micromanage his life. We only wanted to improve his quality of life based on what he had communicated with us about his end-of-life wishes years ago. We knew that our dad did not want to die. We also knew after watching him a number of times that there comes a point where the human body no longer cares what the person wants.

On some level, it is easier to help someone that I am not connected to through family ties make decisions about the end of their life. The emotional and relational investment is less. You may be feeling this way right now. Clients value my insight and experience in ways my parents do not. After my mom died, my dad and I had a direct conversation about his end-of-life wishes. At first, he said, when it came to that point, he would go out of the woods, sit under a big tree, and take care of himself. I continued to press him for what he really wanted. He realized that I was serious about having this conversation, and then he shared his thoughts along with his end-of-life documents. He had made it clear that my stepmom was the one in charge of his health and well-being if he could no longer make decisions for himself. I thought taking those steps was enough to prepare for what was to come. Turns out, it has not been.

My dad has been one of my greatest teachers. He potty trained me, taught me to ride a bike, showed me how to tie my shoes, and he is the voice in my head gently instructing me to pick up that piece of paper on the floor instead of walking by it. It is only fitting that he would also be my biggest teacher in allowing other people to make choices for themselves in the later part of their lives. My father and I are in agreement when it comes to what is written on his legal end-of-life documents. They are full of clear instructions that are easy to follow. But my dad is not actively on his deathbed; he is living the last part of his life, and his fragile medical status means that it is not going to plan. I have to be okay with that because the human body is going to what it will based on the life the person is leading.

As humans, our physical bodies do not function independently from our environment or the daily choices the individual makes. This statement is not meant to place blame on an individual for their body's behaviors at the end of life. Blaming does not help. People make all types of decisions for all kinds of reasons that may be unknown to the person sitting at the bedside. My sister and I informed our dad after his last major hospital stay that it was time to move into a facility so he could have a higher quality of life by being managed medically by professionals. Our family came to an agreement that this would be the plan. As soon as my dad started gaining mental clarity at the rehab facility, my stepmom and I began talking about his coming home.

While I am a big advocate for aging in place and dying at home, I also understand that both of these things can be done better with proper support and home setup. My parents wanted no outside professional help, and their house was not set up to support someone with my dad's health issues. That has been proven time and time again with their firing home health care aides and turning down my offers to update things around the house.

Why am I sharing all of this with you? Trust me, it is not just because I need to vent. It is because it has been my greatest lesson as an advocate for ensuring that people at the end of life are allowed to have a voice in what is happening to them. I do not agree with many of the decisions my parents are making about the last part of my father's life. My views on when to step into their lives with professional guidance and offers of help have changed. You cannot give people what they don't want. My dad and stepmom do not want my professional guidance. They want the version of me that is their daughter, not a death doula. While I cannot separate my training from who I am, I practice restraint while following their lead. I allow my parents to be fully human and to make decisions for themselves, even when I do not like them. Unless they are making an unsafe choice, they are in control of their lives.

I bring my awareness of allowing another person agency and autonomy at the end of their life to you as you sit at the bedside of your loved one. You may not agree with the lifestyle choices that brought them to this point. You may not agree with the types of support they have chosen to have at the end of their life. You may be mad about or exhausted by what they did not properly plan for. You may want to blame them, their medical team, yourself, or some other person for your loved one's dying time. Blaming someone for what is happening at the moment is easy, and it can protect you from your true feelings, but in the long run, it can be detrimental.

PAUSE AND REFLECT EXERCISE: Emotional Release

Create space to acknowledge difficult emotions without being consumed by them.

Purpose: To recognize and express challenging feelings in a safe way, reducing their power and creating emotional breathing room.

Time needed: 3-5 minutes in a private moment

Instructions:

1. Take a moment to slow down and acknowledge your current emotional experience.
2. Notice what feelings are present—perhaps anger, resentment, sadness, guilt, or apathy.
3. Allow these emotions to simply be without pushing them away or judging them.
4. Check in with your body: Where are you feeling tension or discomfort related to these emotions?
5. Remind yourself that these feelings don't need to take over or define you.
6. Take a deep breath if that feels comfortable.
7. Look up at the ceiling for a moment, creating physical and mental space.
8. Allow yourself to express what you're feeling, either silently or aloud: "I hate this," "I wish this were different," or "I feel..."
9. Let the words come without censoring, giving yourself permission to feel what you feel.
10. Notice any sense of release as you express these emotions honestly.
11. Take another deep breath, observing how your emotional landscape may have shifted.
12. Remind yourself that you're not trapped by the situation or by your feelings about it.

Reflection: How did naming your emotions affect their intensity? What changed in your body after this brief exercise? Does creating this emotional space help you return to caregiving with more presence?

Another thing I have learned as a death doula is that in between planning for the end of life and actually reaching the end of life, there is a gap filled with uncertainty. The later stages of life can be short or can extend for years. That time period can be full of quality shared experiences and stressful caregiving. The first thing you can do in the gap between having end-of-life planning conversations and reaching end-of-life is to honor the gap and the unknown. I think one of my unconscious reasons for becoming a death doula was that I would have training that provided me with tools and techniques to deal with my loved one's dying times. It offered me a measure of control. What I am learning from my father is even with extensive training, supporting someone at the end of life while honoring their wishes can be challenging. In my years of experience, I've learned that those at the bedside look for things to control in what feels like an uncontrollable situation. Sitting at the bedside of a beloved person, watching them die, can make you feel out of control like you have been removed from the world and teleported to a different place where time goes weird.

Think about when the pandemic started, and no one knew what was happening or how long we would be locked down. What did a number of people rush out and do? Buy toilet paper. Why? Because of so many unknowns, people reach for a level of certainty that can be found in stocking up on toilet paper. Another example of this is when a major weather event, like a snowstorm, is about to take place. Anytime a big storm is predicted, people go to the grocery store and buy essentials- sometimes even if they do not need them. Daily, we operate as though we are in total control of our lives, but much remains out of our purview, and acknowledging that thought can be scary. So, what do you do when you are faced with a situation that leaves you feeling powerless? You reach for what you can trust, for the things that feel tangible- you have the conversations about end-of-life planning, and you try to follow those plans as best you can, all while being kind and patient with yourself because honestly, no one knows how this journey with your loved one is going to go. In accepting the unknown, you allow space for what may come up.

There is a belief that at the end of life, the dying person's brain takes them through a life review. This "flash before your eyes" moment gives the person a chance to go over the highlight reel of their life. It is thought that it happens quickly. But what about the person at the bedside?

PAUSE AND REFLECT EXERCISE: The Relational Tapestry Check-In

Take time to notice how your relationships are shifting during this journey.

Purpose: To create space for acknowledging your emotions and insights about changing relationships during this challenging time.

Time needed: 5-10 minutes in a quiet moment

Instructions:

1. Take a deep breath, and give yourself a moment to think about your journey with your loved one.
2. Remember that insights often unfold gradually—there's no need to rush this process.
3. As you sit with the reality of their end-of-life

journey, pause to ask yourself: What stands out most for you right now?

4. Notice what emotions are present: Frustration? Disappointment? Gratitude for support? Numbness?
5. Remind yourself: There's no right or wrong way to feel—only your way.
6. Consider how the relationships in your life weave together into a complex tapestry of experiences.
7. Reflect on how those connections are shifting and changing during this time.
8. Ask yourself:
    - What do you notice about your relationship right now?
    - What are you learning about yourself and your loved one?
    - Which threads in your relational tapestry feel tight, and which ones are loosening?
9. Give yourself permission to feel whatever arises without judgment.

Reflection: How does pausing to recognize these relationship shifts help you navigate this time? What patterns do you notice in how you respond to these changes?

~

In my mother's dying time, loosening these knots of control was easy. The time from her terminal illness diagnosis to the end of her life was short. We had already been estranged, which led me to loosen some of the connections I had with her. Add to all that, the decisions that my mom made during her dying time were ones that I agreed with. It's easier to allow a person to make their own choices if you agree with them. Now, in contrast to the relational tapestry I weaved with my father. My dad is not actively dying. Although his fragile health has brought him very close to death many times. While my mother was my greatest inspiration in becoming a Death Doula, my father is my greatest test and practicing the art of allowing someone to make their own choices at the end of life.

9

UNDERSTANDING PHYSICAL CHANGES

In this chapter, I will cover bodily changes that may occur for your loved one and the physical parts of dying. I will also discuss some of the unusual, unexplainable things that might take place during your loved one's dying time. First, though, I want to cover something that few people who have supported a loved one at the end of life may have shared with you. That is the many losses that happen before your loved one takes their last breath. You see, long before someone leaves this world, they are faced with other losses- such as the loss of the idea that they have unlimited time left to live, the loss of confidence in their bodily strength, and the loss of a future. Almost daily, your loved one may be faced with changes that cause them to come to grips with what they no longer have and accept a new reality as they release from their physical being.

At the same time, those at the bedside are faced with losses. Maybe no one has mentioned to you how grief can take hold before someone dies. When you first heard about your loved one's diagnosis or saw how their body was beginning to show less vitality, how did you feel? How did you react? Before becoming a death doula, I remember how it was for me. I felt as though I had been punched in the gut. I remember moments of anger and confusion. My emotions punched a hole in my heart, allowing me to realize that what I was feeling was loss. Ultimately, what I felt was grief. Even when my family members were still alive, I felt the loss of how they had moved about in their lives when they were healthy. I still have a photo that sums up this part of my grandfather's dying journey. In it, my dad and my grandfather are walking around the backyard of my grandparent's house, where my grandmother's rare trees thrive. The men pictured holding hands, a gesture they had not done a few years prior. Their hand-holding demonstrated the strong love that they felt for each other, and the gesture was necessary. My dad, who had never been as big or strong as his dad, was now the stronger and bigger one; they held hands because my grandfather was no longer able to walk unassisted and was thin and frail. The photo is beautiful and heartbreaking all at once. It is full of love and also evidence of everything that was missing from that moment in time. Later, when my Grandpa Lee was in hospice at home, I was grateful to still see his smile but missed his strong hugs and his big presence standing in the room. During my mother's dying time, which was much swifter, I recall my immense feelings of loss with all of the changes my mom experienced. Just as I had come to terms with my mom's new normal, another change would take place. First, her cancer diagnosis knocked me over, then my fiercely independent mother's ability to live on her own went away, and just as her body was growing weak enough that she needed a walker, she died. Adding to the grief that I felt over all my mother's physical limitations and needs was the grief I felt over our relationship and how it had not always been great. Our exchanges during my mother's dying time were colored by the complicated nature of our relationship. We missed the good moments in our time as mother and daughter, knowing that we could never live those times again. We missed what we were not able to have during the years that we fought. Not every change was as hard as some for me, but the one that was the most difficult was hearing my mom grappling with her own mortality.

One of the toughest things about supporting a loved one during their dying time is that your needs and emotions often take the backseat to what they need. Logistically, that becomes almost necessary for many people acting as caregivers. How could you continue to support a dying person while feeling the immensity of the experience? I have talked to many people who have said that during their caregiving journey, they could not open themselves up to their true feelings because they were afraid that the rush of emotions would be too much. It would interfere with their ability to take care of their loved one's needs. Even if you are not your loved one's primary caregiver, if you are sitting at the bedside with them, it can be difficult to allow yourself to grieve what has changed. After all, you have a life going on outside of the dying space, and not everyone will be compassionate or patient with you. Most likely, though, you will be the one who has the least amount of compassion and patience for yourself.

The thing is that your loved one's dying and your experience of that are, in fact, happening at the same time. While you do not have to spend hours reflecting on how you feel at this moment, you can give yourself a few seconds to let your heart catch up with what your eyes see. I love death doula Dr. Sarah Kerr's teaching on how time is interpreted when supporting the dying. Dr. Kerr talks about soul timing and how our brains register events faster than our hearts and our beings can process them. Give yourself time to acknowledge what you are going through, even if it means looking at the ceiling and thinking about how hard this all is for twenty seconds or taking a deep sigh while not really thinking about anything at all. Don't worry about how to do it. Just when you are feeling strong emotions, whether it be frustration, exhaustion, or grief, give your heart a few moments to catch up with your thoughts.

Even though I just said not to worry about how to discharge or find ways to accept your feelings, at the end of the book, I have included resources where you can find exercises to utilize when you need support.

Now, I am going to begin to cover the phases of dying and the physical changes that can occur during the end of life. If you are not comfortable learning about this material, skip it. The information provided is uncomplicated and rational, but that does not mean it will be easy to read, considering what you are going through.

Dying can be broken up into stages. There is an early, middle, and late stage, also known as active dying. Every stage in the dying process is marked by changes in the body's ability to function and the individual's responsiveness. Remember, the experience of dying varies from person to person, and not everyone progresses through the stages the same way. It can even be the case that stages are passed through quickly enough that the smaller shifts in physical functions are not noticed.

The early stage of dying can last anywhere from one month to three months before death. During this phase, people often experience decreased appetites, increased sleepiness, heightened pain and nausea, visible weight loss, reduced activity levels, and ambivalence toward their surroundings. During this stage, a dying person can be at higher risk for developing infections. There might also be emotional changes that cause a person to withdraw, decrease their level of communication with others, and become more introspective.

The middle stage of dying can range from weeks to days. Signs of this stage of dying include extreme fatigue, confusion, and more pronounced social withdrawal. A few days before active dying begins, people may experience an intensification of emotional and physical symptoms. The individual may also experience difficulty swallowing, which can lead to breathing sounding different due to saliva collecting in the back of a person's throat. Symptoms in all stages of the dying process can be managed medically, physically, spiritually, and/or psychologically to varying degrees. If your loved one experiences any changes that are concerning to you, please ask their hospice or medical team for support. It is their job to help your loved one, and part of that is helping you when you have questions or concerns.

The active stage of dying begins two to three days before death. Common symptoms during this phase include breathing changes, significant drops in vital signs such as blood pressure, and increased unresponsiveness. A person in this stage may let their head droop to one side, their mouth may remain open, and their skin color may change. In the last part of the active dying stage, an individual may experience periods where they stop and restart breathing. The dying person's eyelids may remain open, and they may grunt due to vocal cord tension. If you suspect that this is due to pain, tell your loved one's medical team. In all stages of dying, the body undergoes metabolic changes that help the person die. While the changes you see during your loved one's dying may seem out of the ordinary to you, to the hospice and medical personnel, it probably seems normal. Do not be afraid to ask them about things that seem abnormal to you.

Now that I have covered the stages of dying and what

your loved one might experience, I am going to provide you with some further explanations about physical changes and what you can do to support your loved one during these changes.

COMFORT LEVEL CHANGES

Discomfort during a person's dying time can come from a variety of sources. Pain is just one of them. The goal of pain management is to lower discomfort to tolerable levels. Removing all pain may not be possible, but at the end of life, medical providers can give higher doses of medications to alleviate pain without worrying about long-term problems of drug dependence. Nobody gets the label of a drug addict at the end of life. If you suspect your loved one is experiencing unmanaged pain, then contact their medical team ASAP. Never fear telling your loved one's providers that they might be in pain. Prevention of pain is easier than relieving pain. Severe pain symptoms can be hard to manage, so it is a good idea to know what clues to watch for that indicate your loved one is in pain. Know, though, that not everyone experiences pain at the end of their life.

Clues that your loved one may be experiencing pain include trouble sleeping, increased agitation, and crying. They may reach or touch a painful area. I remember during my grandma Jan's dying time how, even though she was not conscious, my grandmother put her hand on her side where a previous treatment had been. I knew she was in pain and told her nurse. My grandmother was able to relax and stop holding her side after the nurse gave her medicine. Another sign of pain may be a slight change in facial expression. Furrowing the brow, grimacing the face, or clenching the jaw can indicate that your loved one is feeling discomfort. You know what your loved one's expression is normally. Watch for any changes in how they look based on your experience of them.

Discomfort can also be caused by breathing problems and skin irritations, including itchiness, digestive problems, temperature sensitivity, and fatigue. When a person is uncomfortable in the dying process, they do not just lie there. They will be restless, and they may make noises. They will show those at the bedside that they are uncomfortable through body language. In the following paragraphs, I will cover some of the other changes that you may see and offer a few tips on how you may be able to manage them.

BREATHING CHANGES

Shortness of breath or difficulty in breathing is common at the end of life. Some terms that the medical team may use when discussing breathing issues during the dying process are Cheyne Stokes breathing, which is when a person alternates between deep, heavy breaths and shallow breathing. There can even be a pause in breathing. This breathing pattern can be hard to watch at the bedside. Remember to not hold your breath too much while watching your loved one's breathing patterns.

The death rattle is noisy breathing usually caused by the saliva collecting in the back of the individual's throat. The dying person is generally relaxed enough that this is not uncomfortable for them, but it can be hard to listen to

Agonal breathing is gasping for air. If it happens, it is usually at the very end of a person's life. The person who does this type of breathing is usually no longer conscious or aware of what is going on. Their brainstem is trying to keep their body full of oxygen even though their body is actively shutting down. It is a normal bodily response for the central nervous system to trigger this type of breathing. If this breathing pattern becomes worrisome, contact your loved one's medical provider. Agonal breathing usually does not last long, but it can be difficult to sit with a person who is breathing this way.

What you can do to help ease breathing troubles such as shortness of breath is to raise the head of your loved one's bed or bolster them up with additional pillows. You can also open a window, use a humidifier, or use a fan to circulate air in the room. If your loved one is willing, meditation or breathing exercises may help with difficulties.

SKIN CHANGES

Skin color changes that occur during the dying process are usually due to decreased circulation of blood, which results in low oxygen levels in the body. The kidneys also slow down, which can lead to color changes. Depending on your loved one's normal skin color, their skin could become yellowish, whitish, purplish, pale grey, greenish, or bluish. They may also experience blotchiness, especially on their hands or feet. Their fingertips can show signs of decreased circulation by becoming paler. A dying person's sensations in their arms or legs may also decrease. They may experience numbness. Your loved one may also show signs of swelling, especially in the arms and legs, because of the decreased fluid movement in the body. Skin problems can be uncomfortable for someone going through the dying process. Keep your loved one's skin clean and moisturized by using alcohol-free lotions. This can help relieve itching and dryness. Dryness of the face and mouth can become a problem for your loved one. Keep their lips moist with lip balm and their mouth clean with a soft, damp cloth. For dry eyes, you can gently apply non-irritating eye cream or gel around their eyes. You always have the option of placing a damp cloth over their eyes to keep them closed.

It is important to watch for bed sores if your loved one has been bed-bound for a long period of time. Even if they have not been in bed for long, certain medical conditions can lead to the skin breaking down easily. To prevent skin breakdown, try to reposition your loved one every few hours. This may also help them with any stiffness they experience. You can always use foam pads or extra pillows to cushion their heels or elbows to help reduce pressure on those bony areas. Honestly, there will be a point in your loved one's dying process where repositioning may seem silly or disruptive to their rest. Trust your ability to decide if they need to be moved.

TEMPERATURE CHANGES

When a person is going through the dying process, they may experience a wide range of temperature changes. One person may experience feeling cold when they are dying. Another person may feel hot and get sweaty. A person who is nearing death may have hands, feet, arms, and legs that are cool to the touch. This may be associated with them feeling cold, and then again, it may not. Your loved one may not be able to tell if they are hot or cold. A sign to watch for that can be attributed to overheating is agitation. If your loved one is overheated, they may continually throw off their covers. If this happens, remove the covers, maybe offer them a sheet to cover up with if needed, and try placing a cool, damp cloth on their forehead. A sign to watch for to see if a person is cold is shoulder hunching, pulling covers up, and shivering. If your loved one gets cold, they may feel increased pain.

DIGESTIVE CHANGES

Toward the end of a person's life, it is normal to see decreases in appetite. If your loved one no longer has the desire to eat or drink, do not force them to do either. You can continue to gently offer your loved one small amounts of the favorite or other easily digested snacks like apple-sauce, but know your loved one may decline the offer. I remember watching the author Elizabeth Gilbert speaking about attending her partner's end of life. All her partner wanted to eat was Oreos. Elizabeth did not fight her girl-friend on this. She knew her love was dying, so she let her eat whatever she could tolerate- cookies. Your loved one may find a specific item more appetizing than other food. Trust your intuition and follow their lead on eating. For dry mouth, offer your loved one ice chips if they are still conscious and able to swallow. Swallowing can become difficult at the end of life, which can contribute to a decreased desire to eat and drink. You can use a straw to offer drops of water in their mouth if your loved one is unable to drink from a cup or has difficulty swallowing larger amounts of liquids. Mouth swabs provided by hospice can also be used to alleviate dry mouth and provide the caregiver with a sense of offering nourishment to their loved one. The metabolic changes happening in the body during the dying process reduce the need for food and liquids. Going without food or water at the end of life is generally not painful. In fact, eating and drinking can add to a dying person's level of discomfort.

Nausea, vomiting, and constipation can occur during a person's dying time. This may be due to the pain meds your loved one is taking. It can also be a natural part of the body's process of shutting down the digestive system. Talk to your loved one's medical team about any symptoms you see that are problematic. Practitioners may be able to offer treatments to help ease symptoms.

ENERGY LEVEL CHANGES

It is common for people at the end of life to be tired and to have low energy levels. It is also common for caregivers to experience fatigue. What you and your loved one are going through is challenging. It can be exhausting work for all involved.

Any fatigue that your loved one experiences could have physical causes or psychological causes. When the body's processes begin to slow down, it becomes hard for it to accomplish its basic functions. Add to that the feelings and emotions that your loved one may have, and it is natural that they may experience fatigue. It is also normal for someone at the end of life to experience anxiety or depression. There are medications that can be given to help with this if your loved one wants to take them, but know that they have a right to feel the way they do. The same goes for you. There are medications that you can take to help you psychologically through this time, and you have the right to take them or to say no thanks to them. Your loved one's doctor or licensed mental health provider can help you both decide what is best for them. Same for you. If you are struggling with your mental and physical energy, your physician and/or mental health provider can help you decide if you could benefit from medication.

Restlessness and agitation can increase in your loved one, and in addition to having physical causes, they can be caused by emotional and mental distress. It is not uncommon for someone going through the dying process to have wandering attention, outbursts, aimlessness, or show strange behaviors that appear suddenly. These can be caused by physiological changes in the body, such as decreased lung function and decreased kidney function. They can also be caused by medications in addition to increased levels of pain.

Mental energy and physical energy are connected. If your loved one feels poorly physically, there is a good chance they may not feel great mentally and vice versa. Humans have a strong mind-body connection, even if we are unaware of it. Talking with someone about what your loved one is experiencing may benefit them. This also applies to you. The listener does not have to be a professional. There are certainly numerous professionals- counselors, chaplains, psychiatrists, coaches- who are trained to help, but talking to a friend or family might be enough. The benefit of talking to a professional is that it is their job to listen, and they may not be as emotionally burdened by the shared information as a family member or friend might be. Either way, having the knowledge that there is help when your loved one or you need it can offer benefits. You do not even have to get help to receive the benefits. Just knowing it is there can support you.

One other energy change that can take place with a dying person is a surge in energy. This can be referred to as a life surge or a sunset day. A life surge can occur days, hours, and even minutes before a person dies. This surge can offer a few moments in which your loved one may experience increases in alertness, have more energy, and have a clearer mind. This rally in energy can be confusing because it can appear that your loved one is improving when they are actually not. Not every person at the end of life experiences a surge in energy. If your loved one does, then take advantage of this gift. If your loved one does not experience this, know that they and those around them did nothing to prevent it from happening. It is not exactly clear why a life surge takes place, and it cannot be predicted.

As your loved one gets closer to the end of their dying

process, their healthcare team may check their vital signs less often. They do this to allow your loved one more undisturbed rest. If your loved one is dying in a hospital or facility, some monitors may be silenced or removed. You can always request more or less interaction from their team. If your loved one is at home, there is a chance that their healthcare will not be present for large portions of their dying time. Most hospice services have numbers you can call with any concerns you have. Hopefully, you will have the same nurse or a couple of nurses visiting your loved one so the relationship can be established.

DEATHBED PHENOMENA

At your loved one's end of life, there is the possibility that transcendent phenomena may take place. In this book, I am not going to tell you that what your loved one and you see or experience is or is not real. When people share stories about deathbed phenomena with me, I tell them that it is not anybody's place to tell them if it was or was not real. I call anything that falls into the category of deathbed transcendent phenomena or coincidences the unknown of the dying process.

It is not a secret that there are mysteries around the dying process. When you attend the bedside of a dying person, you have to release your grip on certainties and be open to shifts and uncertainties that may occur during a person's dying time. Any number of shifts can occur during your loved one's dying journey. Then again, nothing strange or out of the ordinary may take place.

Some of the phenomena that I am aware of include deathbed visions. This is where the dying person sees things, people, or pets that are not physically in the room. In my experience, this is usually a positive experience for the dying person. The only time I have witnessed it not be positive was with my own grandmother. As my sister and I sat with her, our grandmother's room grew cold, and she started waving her hand and saying, "Go away. Not now." Our grandmother repeated this a few times, calmed down, and then the room warmed back up. My sister and I looked at each other to see if we had the same experience. We did. Our grandmother died the next morning before we arrived at her bedside. This story not only demonstrates that dying people can experience visits from people who passed away before them but also that a dying person may choose who they want to be present with in their last moments. I have no scientific proof for this if you are looking for it. I only have anecdotal evidence, personal experience, and others' stories.

Another occurrence that can take place is the dying person or a recently deceased person visiting someone who is not present in the dying space. Karen, a grief client of mine, told me about how her sister, Darlene, who was in ICU in a hospital states away, visited Karen in a meditation a week before Darelene died to let Karen know she was releasing from her body. Then, on the day of Darlene's death, their older sister, who was at the bedside, said that Darlene opened her eyes and squeezed the other sister's hand before dying. I explained to Karen that there are mysteries that surround the dying process, and maybe Darlene showed up to say goodbye in her dying time in ways that she knew each sister could comprehend. The way our perception works and how time is experienced can become weird when someone you love is dying.

The phenomena of seeing light can take place during a person's dying time. This light can fill the entire room, it can emanate from the dying person, it can be a shape that moves about the space... I have heard many stories of light showing in numerous ways. I have also experienced this myself.

As a person gets closer to the end of their dying time, they may begin to reach out, as though they are reaching for someone or something that is there for them. It can be the case that as words decrease, hand movement increases to express what cannot be spoken. Not only can words be replaced by movements, but the type of language a dying person uses can change. People at the end of life often begin to speak in metaphors. Some phrases that may show up may pertain to a person going on a journey, seeing visitors, finding boxes to hold things, talking about completeness or wholeness, and announcements of big events like parties taking place on specific days in the future. Dying people can also become repetitive in what they say. Their conversations can become a word salad. They can talk about feeling gratitude or feeling reassured. Sometimes, people talk about feeling movement, like being on a train or a boat; they can speak about the vision of crowds present in space, and they can focus on shapes or numbers. Changes in language patterns and conversation topics during a person's dying time are normal. There is no need to correct them if they say something that makes no sense, like seeing a visitor who is not physically present. It can be unnerving if you are with someone who starts speaking unusually or talks about things you cannot see, but it is normal behavior.

Your mind finds comfort in knowing that one explanation of these changes in verbal language and the increase in hallucinations could be due to changes in the dying person's brain chemistry. It is possible that these changes are also the result of the individual's mind creating ways to provide comfort as they near death. Concerning phenomena witnessed by caregivers or those present with the dying, it could be viewed that the unknown events happen in response to the stress of the event. Cultural beliefs can also influence what is perceived at the end of someone's life.

Whatever your loved one and your experience, my words to you are to take what is helpful from the information I provided. If I were there in person, I could guide more on what is being experienced. But no matter whether I guide you in person or through a book, I would tell you to trust yourself first. No one needs to validate your experience. If you need someone to share with who is open to your experience, find a person who is not closed off to the mysteries that can take place at the end of life.

PART IV

THE THRESHOLD AND BEYOND

10

FINAL DAYS

You did not choose this. No one asked if you wanted to add living through the end of your loved one's life to your calendar of events. But here you are. Here your loved one is. Remember, you are human. You are not choosing to support your loved one at the end of their life as a job. You are doing this out of love and maybe necessity. Be kind to yourself. Be patient with yourself. Whether you are the primary caregiver for your loved one or you are spending time with them during their dying time, this is one of the hardest things you will ever do. It asks a lot of you.

It is my belief that how you experience your loved one's dying time will color how you move through the grieving process after they die. In school and in our daily lives, we are taught very few ways to do uncomfortable things. Attending to a dying person can be uncomfortable. For many of us, how to do this is unfamiliar. It can bring up a range of feelings and emotions. It can cause you to reevaluate your relationship with the dying person in good ways and in challenging ways.

Watching your loved one move through their dying journey pulls on the invisible threads that connect the two of you. The physical attachments you have to each other are stretched and eventually cut, leaving only memories and bonds that stretch across time. Sometimes, those bonds are not tight. Whether you have a strong relationship with your loved one or a troubled one, going through their dying time can be taxing. You may even find that you feel nothing at all. Do not shame yourself for how you experience this time.

Supporting your loved one during the time they have left to live requires you to open your heart, show up with a compassionate presence, be attentive, and appear fearless when you are full of uncertainty. What this book is teaching you and asking you to do is to be a comforting presence for your loved one and those in the dying space, to provide a sense of grounding for yourself and others, and to respect that death is something that cannot be outrun. Death doulas are comfortable with death. While you do not have to be 100% comfortable with everything your loved one and you are going through, you can find solace in a stabilizing force. Maybe that force is where your faith lies, maybe it rests in another person in your life, maybe you find it in this book, or maybe sometimes the stable force is inside of you. Most likely, you will call upon a wide range of sources for security and stability during this taxing time. That is okay. You do not always need to have everything together when supporting your loved one. Sometimes things will fall apart, sometimes you may cry, sometimes you may feel nothing at all, and sometimes your loved one may have a bad day.

What you will do is let your loved one know that you will continue to be present for them in whatever ways you decide to support them. You do not even have to speak this; you can show it in your actions. You also will want to continue allowing space for yourself, even when there is no time and you are exhausted. Find a way to at least take five minutes to be who you were before your loved one started their dying journey. Don't lose the entirety of who you were before, and try to be open to growing through this experience. It will change you. There is duality in supporting someone at the end of life. The experience can completely overwhelm you, causing you to be unable to deal with your everyday life and what is required of you in the dying space. The experience can also open you up to a deeper understanding of love and life. Psychotherapist and author Francis Weller says that where there is grief, there is also love. I amend this slightly by saying where there is grief in the dying space, there are strong emotions, love possibly being one of them. It is possible that you find yourself caring for a family member with whom you have a complicated relationship. You may feel obligated to be present for your family member. There may also be no other option than you when it comes to supporting the dying person. Whether or not you are in a close relationship with your dying family member, there will most likely be a dynamic tension between your feelings in the present moment and your feelings about the past and the future. I had someone tell me once that they were feeling "all kinds of ways." I think that is a good description of how you may feel while supporting your family members during their dying time.

It is important that you devote a little energy to taking care of yourself. By taking care of yourself, you provide yourself with the strength to endure the fatigue that may make you question yourself and not trust your intuition. By not taking care of yourself, your unattended needs or feelings may find someone to project themselves onto- whether it be your spouse, your children, your co-workers, or even your loved one. The needs and feelings that you are not dealing with may not come out exactly how you are experiencing them. Your unacknowledged and repressed feelings will find a way to the surface-maybe not now, but eventually. You may find, as my client Greg found when his mom was dying, that other relationships outside of the dying space become strained due to the stress you are dealing with. When Greg's mom entered hospice, he began fighting with his wife. While there may have been other things in their marriage that caused them to fight, the feelings around his mom's end of life intensified Greg's responses. I, myself, experience this when my dad's health puts him in the hospital or my stepmom complains about issues I have offered to help with. You do not live in a vacuum. What affects you in one area of your life may carry over to another. Awareness of this can help you to share with the people you have relationships with, as your patience might be short, you may be more sensitive, or your overtiredness may make you respond in harsh ways. Hopefully, the people around you will have patience and compassion for you. Often, just sharing that you are under pressure will help you to interact in healthier ways with others because it removes the expectation that everything is normal. Unless you serve dying people as your career, what you are doing is not normal. Even for me as a death doula, being with a dying family member puts pressure on me that I do not have when I am working with a client.

There is no right or wrong way to live through the experience of supporting a loved one at the end of their life. There is only what is right at the moment. Sometimes, there is time and energy to consciously choose what is right, and other times, there is only space to respond to what is in front of you. When you resource yourself with tools, techniques, and a general understanding of the dying process, like what is taught in this book, the time and energy available for you to respond increases. The emotional load and physical toll you feel may be lessened. Or it might lead you to realize that you need more help.

There are lots of unknowns when it comes to supporting

a loved one at the end of their life. While this book does not provide you with answers to every scenario you may encounter in the dying space, it does offer you an anchor to hold onto and to keep your head above water until you feel strong enough to move forward. When supporting your loved one, you may not do everything one hundred percent right, but you feel better knowing that you did what you could. And that is healing. That is helping.

11

IMMEDIATELY AFTER

Take a deep breath. Maybe place a hand on your collarbone or on your heart to provide self-soothing. You have reached the point where you see the reality that our time on earth is finite. Your loved one's time is running out. Find meaning in whatever time you have left with them. Sing to them. Read to them. Sit in silence with them. I find that at the end of someone's life, I behave the same way I did when I watched over my newborn children, quietly observing the rise and fall of their breath and listening for their gentle noises that provide proof of life. The main difference between the two situations is that in one, I watch the beginning of a life, and in the other, I watch for the end.

As you watch for your loved one's last breath, know that there is no need to rush what happens. If you question whether or not your loved one is actively dying, call their medical team or hospice. Most likely, their providers will have already shared with you what you might expect to see at this stage of the dying process. Paramedics and emergency medical services are trained to save lives. Unless your loved one has a DNR order, they may work to resuscitate your loved one if called.

You may see many things at the end of your loved one's life, all of which are most likely normal and are not causing unnecessary discomfort for them. There are many ways that the discomfort of dying can be managed medically. Use what the healthcare teams have provided to support your loved one at this time. Use the natural sources of comfort you have been offering to your loved one throughout the entire process. As the body shuts down, each organ that stops functioning affects other body systems. The process is not always straightforward or easy for the dying person. Remember, dying is hard work. You have been witness to all the effort your beloved has put in to get to this point. You have been there when their medical team has been supporting them. You have provided care and comfort to them. Continue this even if you feel it is too much to handle.

Sitting at the bedside in the dying space has possibly already affected how you experience the movement of time. It is said that active dying lasts two to three days following a roughly three-week pre-active dying stage. This estimation is just that, an estimation. In my experience with the dying, the world and time begin to feel reduced and also expanded. Hours feel like days, and days feel like weeks. During a person's dying time, I am aware that the perpetual nature of modern life goes on outside the room whether we in the dying space take part in it or not. But the outside world slips away, and my focus and the way I experience time changes. It almost sharpens to land solely on what is truly important, the dying person and those present with them. What I am attempting to put to words is the otherworldliness of what it is to be with someone when they take their last breath. Somehow, it feels bigger than our understanding could allow while feeling totally natural at the same time. The intimacy of being present for the end of another living being's life takes courage. It carries with it a quiet sense of wonder and sadness. It is hard and beautiful at the same time.

As you sit with your loved one, you may feel as though you are holding your breath, so remember to breathe. Exhale the courage and strength out of your body to assist them as they make the final release from their physical form. Inhale the support and the love that they gave you in life to help you carry on after they are gone. Your loved one's body may be mortal, but their love and spirit can continue on in unbounded ways.

When your loved one breathes their last breath, and their heart ceases to beat, know that you were present for them and with them as they reached a point of completion in their lives, but know there can be a sense of continuation at the end of life. It is said that a person dies three deaths. The first death occurs when the physical body ceases to function. The second death occurs when the body rejoins the earth through burial or cremation. The third death happens when a person's name is no longer spoken by the living. The life and essence of your loved one will continue on in you, as will your life in the people you leave behind. We carry the people who came before us in our very cells and in the rituals for honoring them we create. Tell stories about them. Speak their name. Light a candle in their honor at the same time every week. Share them with the world.

One of the first things I ask people to do when I begin doing grief work with them is to introduce their loved ones to me. This idea is foreign to many of my clients. For many of them, they are accustomed to talking about their loved ones in the past tense. With me, I bring their deceased loved ones to the present with us through conversation. This simple conversational act validates the life of my client's loved one and confirms the impact the loss had on them. It simply gives my clients permission to be sad over the death and also to feel the range of emotions they experienced in sharing a part of life with another human being. You do not need me to do this. It is something you can do on your own. The process starts with the following understanding; being at the bedside is not a performative act. It is a gift that leads to the ultimate tradition of accepting that you are worthy enough to access your grief.

Supporting your loved one throughout their dying journey is not a performance. No one is grading how you show up for their dying time. You do not have to support them to prove your worthiness. You came into this world worthy, as did your loved one. You are both worthy of love, support, kindness, connection, sadness, anger, and grief up to the very end. And after. Neither of you has anything to prove. Their death does not have to be some great lesson that they are required to teach, and your participation in their process does not earn you the right to more sorrow. The idea that, as people, we need to validate our values or our feelings is an illusion. Existence is validation enough.

The gift you are giving to your loved one throughout their dying time is being with them as they live out the remainder of their life. They did not need to be perfect over the course of their life in order to receive this support from you. You do not have to be perfect and all-knowing in order to give it. Gifts are meant to be given and received openly. Hopefully, one day, when it is your time, someone will share this gift with you. By sitting at the bedside of your loved one, you also give yourself a gift. It is the gift of allowing yourself to live the fullness of this experience, to dive deep into the weight of supporting your loved one while still floating in the shallows of everyday life. By supporting your loved one at the end of their life, you have already begun the hard work of grieving their death. You have faced the question of what your loved one's end of life is asking of you by being present in the experience.

In the end, you may rely on strategies to keep putting one foot in front of the other to go on with daily living. There may come a point when those strategies fail, and something deeper is asked to be seen. Something more genuine. The grief you feel will reach out, hoping to draw you into the depths of your being where your loved one still exists. The love and grief for your beloved allow them to continue living inside of you even when they are gone from the physical world. In your heart, in your soul, in your stories, in the mannerisms you inherited from them, in your memories... your loved one exists.

12

YOUR GRIEF JOURNEY

What you may find after their death is that one person's death becomes the affair of those left behind. The business of their life is no longer their worry. It becomes yours or someone else designated to close out their life. This can be exhausting work. It can also be a good distraction from your feelings or a way to tap into them with a safe containment barrier. You can direct all sorts of feelings toward bank statements, house deeds, utility notices... But you still have to come home to yourself and give yourself space and a place to express your feelings.

No matter what your beliefs about the afterlife, whether it exists or not, and what it might look like, there is little argument that the community the deceased leaves behind will feel a huge impact. The closer you are to the individual who died, the more life changes when they are physically gone. The more space a person takes up in your life, the deeper those changes will be felt. I am not saying that only those close to the one who died will feel the impacts of their death. That is just not true. Human connection comes in many forms, small and large. I still grieve deeply for one of my husband's friend, who died years ago. This friend introduced me to sailing and made sure I was comfortable on the water. He was not a part of my daily life, but his presence touched mine in a way only he could. I carry the gift of who he was and what he shared with me in those small moments—always. This is a reminder that we never truly know the full extent of how our loved one's life has touched others or who continues to miss them.

After your loved one's death, you will have no choice but to continue on. I cannot tell you with one hundred percent certainty how this next chapter will go for you. You will take as little or as much time off from your life as you can before the world attempts to pull you out of your feelings of loss. You may want to rush back into normalcy in an attempt to hide away from the experience of your loved one's death, to stay safe from the breadth and depth of your emotions. You may grieve for years. You may feel little and try to shame yourself for experiencing it in a way that you think is normal. I am not here to tell anyone that one way is the right way. Sometimes, you may feel strong and carried by those around you. Other times, you may feel as though people in the world are a million miles away while standing right beside you. I can tell you that the time you may need to process the death will most likely not be matched by the world outside you. The pace of our world is not in tune with the soul's time.

Find people or groups who allow you the time and the space to feel the way you do. When someone tries to rush your grief, say thank you and gently place their well-intentioned thoughts somewhere outside of your mind and your heart. If someone tries to slow down your grief, do the same. One person's way of existing after the loss of a loved one is not always right for another person.

Often, those remaining after death are put in a position of comforting those outside the dying person's circle. What that means is the advice and permission given to you by another after the death of your loved one is more about them than it is about you. They may be uncomfortable with the death of your beloved. They may be uncomfortable with how you are coping with the loss. It is not on you to make yourself palatable for everyone in the world. By honoring your true expressions around what you experienced at the bedside and how you are facing the world after your loved one's death, you unconsciously and without effort give permission to others to do the same.

The grief you feel adds another thread to the weave of your tapestry, knitting you closer to your loved one. As Carson McCullers said, "How can the dead be truly dead when they still live in the souls of those who are left behind?'

Just because someone's part of your story has ended, it does not mean that your story has ended. Once you move away from the acute shock surrounding the death of your loved one, try to find a pocket of happiness every day. Maybe that means you notice how good your morning coffee tastes, maybe it means taking a moment to gaze out the window at the way the sun hits the trees, or maybe it means that you take a deep breath and find a touch of happiness in your ability to pause for a moment. Happiness may, for a while, look different as you negotiate this new world without your loved one.

If your daily schedule was centered around caring for your loved one, then give yourself time to adjust to the lack of routine. Even if there is a celebration of life or a funeral for your loved one, you may find that you are faced with saying goodbye to your beloved every day in the small acts of day-to-day living without them. After a friend of mine's aging dog, Ted, died, I mentioned that he might find himself following the routine that Ted's care had established even though his companion was no longer present. He told me later that he had to take a moment every time he got up from his desk to give Ted lunch or to take his dog outside and allow himself to adjust to this new life without caregiving.

All farewells—whether spoken or silent, expressed through action or stillness—can be seen as gifts, even when they feel overwhelming. But, personal timeline with finding comfort with and the ability to see gifts in a loved one's death is unique to the individual. Research on bereavement is often focused on disruptive grief, which leads to the idea that most people intensely struggle with healing their grief. In actuality, a common reaction to grief is resilience. Grief is highly personal and complex. How one person moves through the grieving process may be different than how another person does. The grieving journey can also vary for a person from day to day.

What this means for you is that the patience and openness skills that you used when supporting your loved one during their dying time will once again be utilized for yourself. Just as you built a community of resources to care for your loved one and to survive their death, you will build a new community of support for yourself.

The resources you will call upon will depend on the structure of your life. Many people find support through their grief journey in peer groups, with friends professionals, and through personal introspection. Just like supporting a dying person relies on layers of support, so does the bereavement process. Recently, I talked with my mother-in-law, Sue, about how she found support after her husband's death decades ago. My father-in-law, Terry, died before I became a part of the family, so I never met him in person. I have, however, met him in spirit through stories shared by family and friends, the resemblances to his dad that my husband carries, and through raising his namesake– my son, Terry. I came to know that my father-in-law took up a lot of space in people's lives and in their hearts, which meant that when he died, the wells of grief ran deep. My curiosity about how my mother-in-law coped with the loss led her to share that although Sue never received professional support, she did unknowingly build a circle of support through her network of friends, neighbors, family members, and church community. This circle held her up and stabilized her footing as she learned to walk through life without her partner's physical presence beside her.

As you move forward in this next chapter in your loved one's dying journey and deeper into your grieving process, take time to pause and reflect on what type of support you may need. You may need to try several avenues of support before finding what feels right. Professionals like myself can offer guidance on how to exist in the world after loss. I work with my clients to help them build a continued relationship with their loved ones now that they are no longer physically present. The work we do together helps them understand the impact of the loss and begins to open a path toward healing.

For now, as you work to build your community of support, know that if you ever find yourself buried beneath emotions, no matter how intense or mild, know that grief is moving through you. I would love to tell you that one day, the grief you feel will be gone, but grief is not something that goes away. Instead, it is something that softens and will become a part of who you are.

Be gentle with yourself. Understand that it is normal to feel all kinds of ways after your loved one's death. It is even normal to feel okay. Do not shame yourself over how you feel. And lastly, after supporting your loved one through the end of their life, remember that there will be times to spread your wings and fly—and times to fold them in and simply be still.

ACKNOWLEDGMENTS

I would like to thank my nephews and niece for being open to receiving my love. I cherish talking to you all. I know you take what you need from our conversations and leave what you don't - just like my readers and clients who take my words and wisdom, filter out what does not serve them, and keep what does. To Leland and Lowell, my first boys, you taught me how to love beyond myself, and you continue to inspire me with your work. To AJ and Johnathan, my second set, you remind me to stay open-minded and hopeful for the future.

The four of you have done great things, and you will continue to do so. My hope is that my work will help you one day if it is needed, just as your presence in the world helps me.

I would also like to thank my early readers- Barbara, Cheryl, and Laurie. Your feedback has been essential to developing my ideas. To my sister Brandi and her husband Billy Joya, your input and support are always spot on. I am honored to share your gifts and presence with the world. For all the people who tell me how great my sister is, I know, and I have known that all my life. Thank you to my sister for marrying someone who would become one of my best friends and biggest supporters. I am forever grateful.

To my kids, Lilly and Terry, thank you for your patience and willingness to let me probe topics that make me feel all kinds of ways. Your hugs and words bring the light back to me. To my husband, Reid, thank you for being an early reader, editing, and encouraging me to keep writing. My hope is that one day, I will see myself as you see me.

Thank you to my wise coworkers in healthcare, to my peers in Human Design, and to all the teachers and clients who have believed in me. And as always, thank you to my parents and the family that came before me. You are the ground upon which I stand.

ABOUT THE AUTHOR

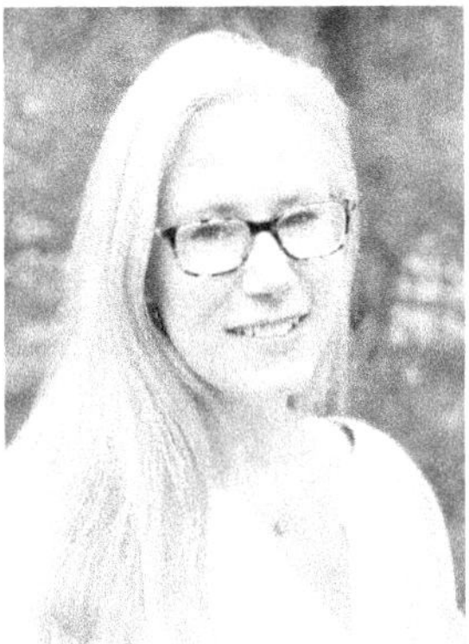

Kelly Ruby Hanson is a Death Doula, surgical technologist, grief educator, and life coach who helps individuals and families navigate their dying and grieving journeys. Raised in a small farming community where multiple generations lived nearby, Kelly grew up witnessing what a good death could look like. After losing several family members as a young adult, she became an advocate for conscious dying and the importance of honoring individual values at the end of life.

Her perspective deepened through years of working in hospitals, where she was present for many deaths, both clinical and personal. After losing her mother, Kelly recognized the limitations of traditional medicine in addressing the emotional and spiritual aspects of loss. She knew she needed a different set of tools to fully support herself and others through the dying process.

Kelly became a certified Death Doula through the Conscious Dying Institute to deepen her work with clients. She now integrates her medical background, practical experience, and education in psychology to guide individuals in being fully present with their loved ones during their final days—and in healing after loss. Her approach blends the language of medicine with psychological insight and holistic practices to help people build strength and resilience in the face of death.

Kelly lives in Colorado and holds a degree in clinical psychology from MSU Denver. She trained in surgical technology through Indiana University, Methodist Hospital, and Riley Hospital and is currently earning a master's degree in social work. In her free time, she enjoys being outdoors, reading, and cooking. Kelly carries with her gratitude for each death she has supported and the lessons those experiences have taught her about living fully and dying openly. She believes that every person deserves to die in alignment with their values, surrounded by those who honor their wishes.

Website: https://www.rubyhanson.com

Email: kelly@rubyhanson.com

Facebook: https://www.facebook.com/Yourlocaldeathdoula

THANK YOU

Thank you for allowing me to be a companion to you in this tender and deeply human work of supporting a loved one at the end of life. Whether you read this book in preparation, in the midst of caregiving, or after your loved one has passed, I hope you found guidance, comfort, and validation in these pages.

Grief is not a problem to be solved—it's a relationship to be honored. If you are now navigating life after loss and are seeking support, I invite you to reach out. I work one-on-one with individuals who are grieving, helping them find meaning, connection, and healing in the wake of loss. Together, we can explore what it means to carry your loved one forward while living fully in your own life.

You don't have to walk this road alone.

To learn more or to connect with me directly, please visit www.rubyhanson.com, connect with me on Facebook at Your Local Death Doula, or by email at kelly@rubyhanson.com.

With gratitude and care,
Kelly Ruby Hanson

PART V

RESOURCES

COPING EXERCISES

COPING EXERCISE: The Fifty-Fifty Awareness Practice

Develop the skill of balanced attention between yourself and your loved one.

Purpose: To maintain awareness of your own internal experience while remaining present and attentive to your loved one, preventing emotional overwhelm while ensuring quality care.

Time needed: 2-3 minutes initially; practice regularly to develop this skill

Instructions:

1. Begin by taking a deep breath and noticing where your body makes contact with its support (chair, floor, etc.).
2. Gently scan your internal landscape, acknowledging any emotions, physical sensations, or thoughts arising within you. Don't try to change them—simply notice.
3. Name these experiences to yourself: "I'm feeling anxious," "My shoulders are tense," "I'm worried about what comes next."
4. Now, with this self-awareness as your foundation, turn your attention to your loved one.
5. Observe them with curiosity and care, noticing their expressions, breathing, positioning, and any cues they may be giving.
6. Continue to maintain this dual awareness—50% attuned to your own experience, 50% attuned to theirs.

7. If you notice yourself becoming overwhelmed by either your emotions or theirs, gently return to your breath and physical sensations as an anchor.
8. Remember: You can be present for someone while still having thoughts and feelings about yourself.

Reflection: How does maintaining awareness of your own experience change how you interact with your loved one? What do you notice about your capacity to be present when you're not trying to suppress your own feelings?

COPING EXERCISE: Self-Witness Practice

Create a moment of present awareness to ground yourself during stressful times.

Purpose: To interrupt automatic patterns of stress and reconnect with your sensory experience, creating a reset point during challenging moments.

Time needed: 1-3 minutes

Instructions:

1. Suspend: Hit the pause button on anything that you are doing.
2. Notice: Observe your environment with attention to each sense:
3. Don't Judge: Track what you observe without judgment. In this moment, there is no good, no bad. There just is.
    - What do you hear in your environment?
    - What do you see in the space around you?
    - Do you smell anything or taste anything?
    - What sensations are present in your physical body?
4. Breathe deeply: Take several conscious breaths before returning to what you were doing.

Reflection: How does this brief pause change your relationship to what you were doing? What shifts in your body, emotions, or thoughts after this simple practice?

COPING EXERCISE: Soothing and Supportive Touch Practice

Use gentle self-touch to calm your nervous system and provide comfort.

Purpose: To ground yourself in moments of stress or overwhelm through intentional, nurturing touch.

Time needed: 5-15 minutes

Instructions:

1. Bring your palms together, noticing the warmth and connection between your hands.
2. Cup your hands in your lap, palms facing up, allowing your body to settle.
3. Move your hands to hover near your heart, feeling the warmth.
4. Gently place one hand on your clavicle (collarbone) area, rubbing or circling with light pressure.
5. Place one hand over the other on your chest, feeling your heartbeat.
6. Use one hand to stroke or make circles on your chest while the other rests.
7. Place one hand on your heart and one on your belly with light pressure.
8. Rest both hands on your belly, feeling the rise and fall of your breath.
9. Place one hand softly on your cheek.
10. Place both hands on each cheek, feeling the warmth.
11. Position one hand on your cheek and one on your forehead.

12. Cross your arms and hug yourself across your chest.
13. Cross your arms and hug around your shoulders.
14. Cross your arms and hug around your belly.
15. Gently stroke your forearms.
16. Return to cupping your hands in your lap.
17. Explore any other gentle touches that feel soothing to you.

Reflection: Which touchpoints felt most calming? How did your body respond to different forms of touch? What changes did you notice in your breathing or tension levels?

COPING EXERCISE: Practicing Presence

Develop the skill of being fully present through mindful seeing.

Purpose: To create a state of non-reactive, nonjudgmental awareness that allows you to be genuinely present with your loved one, even when they cannot fully reciprocate.

Time needed: 5-7 minutes

Instructions:

1. Start by tuning into the awareness of your vision. What do you notice?
2. Focus your eyes on an object in your environment.
3. Allow your eyes to relax and establish a soft-focused view that widens what you see. Tap into your peripheral vision in a way that slightly blurs what is directly in your line of sight.
4. Close your eyes to rest them and allow them to relax. Now, just breathe.
5. Open your eyes without focusing on anything. Soften your gaze and try not to aim your vision at anything.
6. Notice your breathing as you soften your eye sockets.
7. Continue until you feel a relaxation, an ease, or a letting go of your being.
8. Slowly orient your eyes around the room, looking gently while maintaining a soft focus.

Reflection: How does this way of seeing change your experience of your surroundings? What shifts in your body or emotional state when you practice this expansive gaze? How might this presence practice support your interactions with your loved one?

CONNECTION PRACTICES

CONNECTION PRACTICE: A Loving Touchstone

Create a physical object that carries your love and connection.

Purpose: To establish a tangible symbol of your love that can provide comfort and connection for both you and your loved one.

The time needed: 15-20 minutes for initial preparation; ongoing moments of connection

Instructions:

1. Find a smooth, beautiful stone that feels comforting in your hands.
2. Hold it close to your heart, allowing it to absorb your love and energy.
3. As you hold the stone, silently offer all the loving thoughts and feelings you wish to share with your loved one—those tender expressions of care, even the ones that go unspoken.
4. When the time feels right, bring the stone to your loved one's space. If they are able, encourage them to hold it gently in their hands. If not, place the stone on their bedside table.
5. Allow your loved one to hold the stone as often as they desire, feeling the quiet connection it fosters between you.
6. After your loved one has passed, keep the stone close, a tangible reminder of the love you shared.

Reflection: How does this physical object create a connection between you? What emotions arise when you touch the stone? How might this simple object serve as a bridge between you even when words are difficult to find?

CONNECTION PRACTICE: A Blanket of Love and Connection

Create a physical token of connection that provides both comfort and meaning.

Purpose: To create a tangible symbol of love and support that can provide physical comfort and emotional reassurance.

Time needed: Initial setup: 1-2 hours; Ongoing additions: 5-10 minutes per person

Instructions:

1. Find a light-colored blanket or sheet, one that can hold the words of care and connection. You may choose to repurpose one from your loved one's home or your own, allowing it to carry the essence of shared memories.
2. Using fabric markers, invite those who have been a part of your loved one's life to write messages of love, support, and well-wishes on the blanket.
3. As you cover your beloved with this blanket, wrap them in the warmth of the heartfelt words and the kindness of those who have touched their life.
4. As visitors come, encourage them to add their own messages to the blanket, continuing to weave a fabric of compassion and connection.

Reflection: How does this physical object create both comfort and connection? What messages seem to bring your loved one the most peace?

CONNECTION PRACTICE: Recipe Book: Preserving Flavorful Memories

Create a tangible legacy of shared meals and memories.

Purpose: To celebrate your loved one's connection to food and preserve their culinary traditions for future generations.

Time needed: Initial gathering: 1-2 hours; Compilation: 3-4 hours (can be spread over days or weeks)

Instructions:

1. If your loved one has a passion for cooking or a deep connection to food, begin gathering their favorite recipes, whether handwritten, passed down through generations, or from treasured sources.
2. Use this as an opportunity to spark conversation with your loved one and others, reminiscing about the meals and flavors that have shaped their life.
3. Include notes, stories, or special memories that relate to each dish.
4. Compile these into a keepsake book that can be shared with family members.

Reflection: How do these recipes tell the story of your loved one's life? What values and traditions are embedded in these culinary practices?

CONNECTION PRACTICE: Candle Lighting Ceremony

Honoring Connection

Create a ritual that connects those present with those at a distance.

Purpose: To establish a regular practice that honors your loved one and creates a moment of connection for everyone who cares about them.

Time needed: 10-15 minutes weekly

Instructions:

1. Choose a day and time each week to honor your loved one by lighting a candle.
2. This practice can begin while they are still at the bedside, allowing both those present and those unable to be there to participate.
3. As the candle is lit, invite everyone to share something special about your loved one—whether aloud or in quiet reflection.
4. This ritual can continue even after your loved one has passed as a way to keep their memory alive.

Reflection: How does creating a ritual influence your experience of grief? What emerges in these moments of intentional remembrance?

CONNECTION PRACTICE: Host a Living Funeral

Create a celebration of life while your loved one can participate.

Purpose: To allow your loved one to experience the love, memories, and impact of their life while they are still present to receive it.

Time needed: Planning: Several days to weeks; Event: 2-4 hours (or multiple shorter gatherings)

Instructions:

1. Consider hosting a "living funeral" as a way to celebrate your loved one while they are still present.
2. Begin by selecting a venue for the event, keeping in mind what your loved one enjoys in their daily life.
3. The nature of the event can be as simple or elaborate as you wish—tailored to their preferences and interests.
4. If your loved one is unable to leave their current location, choose a time and day for a group of loved ones to visit them.
5. You may want to spread the celebration over multiple days, depending on the circumstances.
6. Be sure to document the event with photos, videos, and written messages.
7. Provide guests with books where they can write messages or memories.

Reflection: What did this experience reveal about your loved one's impact on others? How did experiencing this celebration influence your loved one's perspective on their life?

WRITING REFELCTIONS

WRITING REFLECTION: Grief Journal: A Space for Your Heart's Words

Create a private space to process your emotions throughout this journey.

Purpose: To provide an outlet for exploring feelings that may be difficult to express aloud and to document your experience for later reflection.

Time needed: 5-20 minutes, as often as needed

Instructions:

1. Create a grief journal as a safe, open space where your thoughts, feelings, and experiences can flow without judgment.
2. Begin by writing freely, allowing whatever comes to mind to fill the pages. There's no right or wrong here—whether it's a simple observation or deep, complex emotions.
3. If words feel difficult to find, give yourself permission to scribble or doodle on the page.
4. If free writing doesn't resonate, consider using these prompts:
   - My happiest memory of you is...
   - Something I appreciate about you is...
   - What I miss most about how you were before now is...
   - I am handling your dying time by...
   - What I appreciate about your current care is...
   - What I wish I could change about your current care is...

- What feelings do I have about my loved one's dying time?
- What are my biggest concerns about their dying?
- What are the most important things I would like my loved ones to know about our relationship before they pass away?
- What can I learn from this experience?
- What does this experience make me want to prioritize in my life?
- In what ways can I support my loved one?

Reflection: How does writing change your relationship with difficult emotions? Are there patterns in what brings you comfort or distress?

WRITING REFLECTION: Contemplating the Afterlife

Create space to explore beliefs about what happens after death.

Purpose: To reflect on personal beliefs about the afterlife, regardless of religious background, which can bring comfort and perspective during this time.

Time needed: 5-10 minutes for writing, with additional time for reflection

Instructions:

1. Take a moment to sit with your thoughts and consider what you believe Heaven or the afterlife looks like.
2. This practice can be meaningful for anyone, regardless of religious background, so feel free to reframe the question to explore what you think happens after death.
3. Begin by writing down your thoughts, allowing your ideas to flow freely onto the page.
4. Once you have finished writing, take a moment to read over what you've written.
5. Sit quietly with the words and allow yourself to feel whatever arises from within.

Reflection: Did anything surprise you about your own beliefs? How might these reflections influence how you approach your loved one's spiritual needs?

PAUSE AND REFLECT EXERCISES

PAUSE AND REFLECT EXERCISE: Document Inventory

Purpose: To clarify which documents are complete and which still need attention

Time Needed: 30–60 minutes

Instructions:

1. Gather all existing legal and medical documents.
2. Review the guiding questions above.
3. Create an inventory of what documents are present and what's missing.
4. Record where each document is stored.

Reflection: What surprised you about the document inventory process? Were there any unexpected gaps or concerns?

PAUSE AND REFLECT EXERCISE: Medical Preferences Discussion

Purpose: To explore and document your loved one's medical wishes and concerns

Time Needed: 45–60 minutes, with flexibility for breaks

Instructions:

1. Choose a quiet, comfortable space to talk.
2. Go through the medical questions above at a calm pace.
3. Document responses using your loved one's exact words when possible.
4. Revisit this conversation periodically, as preferences may evolve.

Reflection: What insights emerged from this discussion? Were there any emotional moments, fears, or values that stood out?

PAUSE AND REFLECT EXERCISE: Me-She-We Practice

Explore your emotional patterns and interactions during your caregiving journey.

Purpose: To develop an awareness of your response patterns in different situations, helping you navigate the emotional complexity of end-of-life caregiving with greater self-understanding.

Time needed: 15-20 minutes in a quiet, private setting

Instructions:

1. Reflect on Pleasant Moments
    - Think about a recent pleasant situation. How did you feel emotionally?
    - Notice how your body responded. Were you relaxed? Energized? At ease?
    - Consider interactions with others during this time. What did they say or do? How did they respond to you?
    - How do you typically celebrate or savor these moments of joy or peace?
2. Reflect on Mildly Stressful Moments
    - Shift your attention to moments that were mildly or moderately stressful (not overwhelming).
    - Take a deep breath and notice how your body reacts to stressful situations.
    - What emotions typically arise? Do you become emotionally or physically needy?
    - How did others perceive you during these times? What feedback did they offer?

 - Note any patterns in your physical responses to stress.
3. Bring Yourself to the Present Moment
 - Gently shift your focus to your current experience with your loved one's end-of-life journey.
 - Notice any physical sensations that arise when you think about this experience.
 - Reflect on how others are interacting with you during this time.
 - Are you over-functioning (taking on too many responsibilities) or under-functioning (feeling emotionally drained)?
 - What emotions are present? Note them without judgment.
4. Integrating Insights
 - Consider how these insights can inform how you respond to your loved one's journey.
 - Identify emotional or physical patterns you might want to adjust.
 - Reflect on how you can better support your own needs throughout this process.
 - Consider how to create space for your emotions while maintaining balance.

Reflection: What patterns did you notice across different situations? How might awareness of these patterns help you navigate challenging moments in your caregiving journey? What one small change could you make based on these insights?

PAUSE AND REFLECT EXERCISE: Emotional Release

Create space to acknowledge difficult emotions without being consumed by them.

Purpose: To recognize and express challenging feelings in a safe way, reducing their power and creating emotional breathing room.

Time needed: 3-5 minutes in a private moment

Instructions:

1. Take a moment to slow down and acknowledge your current emotional experience.
2. Notice what feelings are present—perhaps anger, resentment, sadness, guilt, or apathy.
3. Allow these emotions to simply be without pushing them away or judging them.
4. Check in with your body: Where are you feeling tension or discomfort related to these emotions?
5. Remind yourself that these feelings don't need to take over or define you.
6. Take a deep breath if that feels comfortable.
7. Look up at the ceiling for a moment, creating physical and mental space.
8. Allow yourself to express what you're feeling, either silently or aloud: "I hate this," "I wish this were different," or "I feel..."
9. Let the words come without censoring, giving yourself permission to feel what you feel.
10. Notice any sense of release as you express these emotions honestly.

11. Take another deep breath, observing how your emotional landscape may have shifted.
12. Remind yourself that you're not trapped by the situation or by your feelings about it.

Reflection: How did naming your emotions affect their intensity? What changed in your body after this brief exercise? Does creating this emotional space help you return to caregiving with more presence?

PAUSE AND REFLECT EXERCISE: The Relational Tapestry Check-In

Take time to notice how your relationships are shifting during this journey.

Purpose: To create space for acknowledging your emotions and insights about changing relationships during this challenging time.

Time needed: 5-10 minutes in a quiet moment

Instructions:

1. Take a deep breath, and give yourself a moment to think about your journey with your loved one.
2. Remember that insights often unfold gradually—there's no need to rush this process.
3. As you sit with the reality of their end-of-life journey, pause to ask yourself: What stands out most for you right now?
4. Notice what emotions are present: Frustration? Disappointment? Gratitude for support? Numbness?
5. Remind yourself: There's no right or wrong way to feel—only your way.
6. Consider how the relationships in your life weave together into a complex tapestry of experiences.
7. Reflect on how those connections are shifting and changing during this time.
8. Ask yourself:
    - What do you notice about your relationship right now?

    - What are you learning about yourself and your loved one?
    - Which threads in your relational tapestry feel tight, and which ones are loosening?
9. Give yourself permission to feel whatever arises without judgment.

Reflection: How does pausing to recognize these relationship shifts help you navigate this time? What patterns do you notice in how you respond to these changes?

www.ingramcontent.com/pod-product-compliance
Lightning Source LLC
LaVergne TN
LVHW022213200926
848481LV00006B/1950
* 9 7 9 8 3 4 9 5 3 3 6 3 1 *